One Hundred I

If patients can learn about Primary Hyperparathyroidism, then why can't medical professionals?

Primary Hyperparathyroidism (PHPT) is well documented to be a very common endocrine disease, yet many doctors and endocrinologists fail to recognise symptoms, have a poor understanding of which blood tests to request, and even how to understand the results.

Outdated literature and online sites state PHPT causes no, or few symptoms. They were likely written by people who have not experienced first-hand, how debilitating symptoms can be, or they have not witnessed the difference between patients before and after a parathyroidectomy (surgical removal of overactive parathyroid glands/adenomas).

Even people who think they have no symptoms, but were diagnosed with high calcium levels, are amazed after surgery at how much better their quality of life becomes. Many patients are left untreated to suffer for many years from this progressive disease. Patients' families also suffer the consequences.

We would like to set the record straight regarding PHPT, and how it feels to be forced to live with it year after year, whilst knowing there is a surgical cure called a parathyroidectomy, performed by experienced parathyroid surgeons.

The letters in this book were written by members of Hyperparathyroid UK Action4Change, to NHS England, Wales, Scotland, Ireland, Northern Ireland, and RCGP on 15th March 2021, asking for a review of education and practice in primary and secondary care, as well as an urgent review of NICE Guidelines that were first published 23rd May 2019.

The guideline committee largely ignored the recommendations of NHS patients (members of Hyperparathyroid UK Action4Change, and registered stakeholders) in over nine hundred comments submitted during the two public consultations.

The result of their decision is that widespread suffering, and medical ignorance regarding recognition and treatment of primary hyperparathyroidism, continues.

Some hospital laboratories are equally to blame for misdiagnosis. Whilst many labs insist on using EDTA vials to test parathyroid hormone (PTH), fully aware of its necessity for accurate results, other labs are very resistant to change, saying 'well, the difference isn't that much'. The difference is inaccurate blood results. How can that be considered acceptable?

Many hospital labs are actively refusing to test PTH when a calcium result falls within the normal range, even when requested by a GP. Of course, this prevents a diagnosis of normocalcemic primary hyperparathyroidism. More about that in my next book.

Sallie Powell

For everyone suffering from undiagnosed or untreated
Primary Hyperparathyroidism;
'Never Give Up'

with very special thanks to all members of
Hyperparathyroid UK Action4Change
and
HPT UK Medical

Especially the One Hundred marvellous people who
joined this event, wrote and shared their stories, to
Action4Change

A huge Thank You to Mr Shad Khan,
Consultant Endocrine Surgeon, at Oxford University
Hospitals; for believing in us, and curing so many of us; in
many instances where we had no one else who would
give us a chance for a better life.

Thank you to Gill, Mo, Des and Claire, for being
wonderful friends, keeping my spirits up, and always
being there for me.

For my lovely son Jordan; unconditional love as always
Thank you for tolerating my obsession with PHPT

Introduction.

Year after year hundreds of patients like myself, are faced with doctors and endocrinologists who do not understand primary hyperparathyroidism in any or all of its classifications. I'm currently one of 2100 members of a support group which I created in September 2014.

Well actually, it's more than a support group. Hyperparathyroid UK Action4change tries to do exactly what our group name suggests; we want to action for change; to stop misdiagnosis and misinformation from doctors to patients with primary hyperparathyroidism.

Many of us have heard the stories of how parathyroid glands were first discovered by Richard Owen in 1850, in a rhino at London Zoo. There are different variations of that story. Over one hundred and seventy years on, and there are different variations about 'new classifications' of primary hyperparathyroidism too. We believe those classifications have always been there, but think it's likely that they were not, and are still not, understood by many doctors. Why? Well, it makes things more complicated, but if patients can get it, they should too. Right? You would think so.

Many doctors don't appear to want to answer the 'why?' question in the same way that patients do. Maybe they just don't have the answers. We, the patients want the answers, and find them. Many of us are very tired of asking our doctors questions and frustrated at getting excuses, and misinformation in response. It's like walking up an escalator that's going down and it's getting us nowhere fast. For many of us, it is also ruining our lives and further endangering our health.

It's little wonder we feel like we're bashing our heads against a brick wall. Many of us face several battles to get the treatment we need. The first battle is often convincing our GP to refer us to a hormone specialist; an endocrinologist. Once we finally get a referral to an endocrinologist, many of us find they are actually far from being a specialist when it comes to parathyroid hormone and primary hyperparathyroidism. We are told we can't have primary hyperparathyroidism if we don't have osteoporosis or kidney stones. Either our doctors are incapable of reading and understanding NICE guidelines, or the guidelines are misleading for them. At a glance in a seven minute appointment we can see why they might be misleading.

Unless a patient has blindingly obvious hypercalcemia, many patients are told *'Well your calcium isn't 'that high, let's adopt the 'watch and wait approach'*, oblivious to the fact ***'The level of calcium does not determine the severity of symptoms'***. People who do their research about hypercalcemia or primary hyperparathyroidism, go back to their doctors armed with information to plead for an endocrine referral. Of course, they are then labelled as obsessive and often berated for using the internet. Some patients are 'lucky' to have a conceding doctor who agrees to the referral to an endocrinologist. That's the first battle over.

The majority of endocrinologists also seem baffled by primary hyperparathyroidism. Here, the NICE guidelines let patients down once again, as they are told by their 'endo' that their calcium isn't high enough to refer to a surgeon and they will have to wait until their calcium reaches 2.85mmol/L or they get osteoporosis and kidney stones. To us, this is barbaric and cruel. It makes no logical sense for a doctor to want to wait for end organ damage or for their calcium to reach a number seemingly drawn from a hat, before offering intervention to their very poorly patients. It makes no sense either, that the NHS would rather spend huge amounts of money on referrals to other departments for the consequences of untreated PHPT, such as fracture clinics, cardiologists, rheumatologists, A&E and urologists, whilst not only keeping their patients very unwell, but actively contributing to the decline of their patients' health. As many endocrinologist have no clue about normocalcemic PHPT, many will refer patients, even with osteoporosis and/or kidney stones, back to their GP, telling them PHPT can't be the cause because their calcium simply isn't high enough. Many don't consider a 24 hour urine sample to see if their body is excreting excess calcium in their urine.

We go back to our doctors who tell us *'well they're 'the experts, let's review the situation in 6-12 months if you're not feeling any better'*. So we sit in front of them, fighting back tears of frustration, feeling defeated and hopeless, made to feel like we're losing the plot. We know that we won't feel better in six to twelve months. This disease is progressive and the future is only likely to become bleak as far as our health is concerned.

We, the patients know this is all very wrong. We have practically nobody in the medical profession who is prepared to stand up and help us. We have to fight this lonely, frustrating battle by ourselves, supporting each other as best we can, when faced with a brick wall of medical ignorance. Some of us find a way to get over the wall by paying privately for treatment. Those of us who have already been forced out of work, or just don't have the means to pay privately; we just have to 'wait and watch' our bodies, minds, and our lives crumble. It is unfathomable to see this disease destroy the lives of so many who are left feeling worthless in the eyes of their doctors. A question which hardly ever gets answered is **WHY**?

I held a campaign day on 15 March 2021. I asked for some of our members to write to Simon Stevens, the Chief Executive Officer of NHS England, in the hope that he might read their woeful journeys, and realise that many of us need help that is being denied to us.

Surely somebody at the top of the NHS can make enough waves to effect change lower down where patients meet GPs and endocrinologists, who dismiss them and send them away on the basis they don't understand their condition. It is really not helpful to patients or doctors, that the UK Society of Endocrinology state on their site; 'You and your hormones'; '*If hypercalcaemia is caused by primary hyperparathyroidism, this condition can be treated, by an operation to remove the enlarged/overactive parathyroid gland, to rectify the calcium levels in the blood. However, it should be emphasised that this is by no means necessary in every case; indeed in the majority of cases, primary hyperparathyroidism is managed without surgery' ** Update for second edition** One of our members contacted The UK Society of Endocrinology on 11 April 2021 about this, and we were most impressed to hear she had a response on the 7 May. Please read their very positive response at the back of this book.*

For every one of the people who have gotten a referral to an endocrinologist or surgeon from their GP, there are many more people who can't get that referral, because their GP didn't think it was required. These people are generally refused because 'their calcium level isn't high enough' and their doctors have failed to understand that parathyroid hormone needs to be tested from the same blood draw as calcium, to determine a misbalance caused by primary hyperparathyroidism. Often this battle originates at hospital labs who simply refuse to test parathyroid hormone if calcium falls within the normal range. This uneducated decision can have an appalling impact on a patient, leading to misdiagnosis.

I decided if we were going to attempt to raise a red flag about secondary care, by writing to Sir Simon Stevens, we may as well write to Professor Amanda Howe, the president of the Royal College of Practitioners, on the same day. In case those letters get ignored, or shredded, I asked some of our members who wrote them, to send them to me, to publish in this book. Many of their stories are hard to read, hard to believe and even harder to accept, that many of them have been and will continue to be ignored and no action taken by their doctors. I think their stories deserve to be told. The letters published here are by some of our members who gave me permission to publish, because they need to be heard.

For every story told here, there are easily another hundred similar stories in the UK. Here are some of the One hundred letters posted on 15 March 2021 to NHS CEO's in England, Wales, Scotland, Ireland and Northern Ireland, and Professor Amanda Howe of RCGP.

Sallie Powell

Event Letter to Simon Stevens from Hyperparathyroid UK

15th March 2021
Our Ref: SJP/SS-CEO NHS/15-03-21

Dear Sir Simon Stevens,

RE: Action needed by NHS England for recognition and treatment of Hyperparathyroidism

I am writing to you as the Founder/CEO of Hyperparathyroid UK, established in September 2014, to ask you to read this letter and others being sent to you today from some of our members. We have three issues to raise;

- The scale of misdiagnosis and misinformation to patients with primary hyperparathyroidism (PHPT), by many consultants, including endocrinologists, throughout the NHS, which causes prolonged treatment delays and can cause harm. We recognise the root is poor education at many levels throughout the NHS.
- We request an immediate update to the NICE guideline for PHPT, published 23 May 2019; https://www.nice.org.uk/guidance/NG132 to help many patients excluded by them based on calcium levels. We consider them to be a failure and that they appear to have been engineered to steer patients away from the NHS, and towards private care with their prohibitive surgical restrictions.
- Immense waste of NHS resources led by poor knowledge of PHPT. To quote Mr Shad Khan, Consultant Surgeon at Oxford University Hospitals; 'Studies looking at the cost effectiveness of parathyroidectomy compared to medical management show that surgery is far superior economically overall; https://www.surgjournal.com/.../S0039-6060(16.../fulltext

In 2016 we wrote to Sir Bruce Keogh to ask him to initiate the process of commissioning NICE guidelines for PHPT. We were grateful he obliged. We became registered stakeholders. Sadly, the guideline committee failed to consider the comments and evidence our members (NHS patients) submitted during the public consultations. The result of those omissions contribute to devastating impacts on patients, which can result in A&E admissions. The important information they omitted;

- Information relating to two classifications of PHPT; normocalcemic PHPT and normohormonal PHPT. Both classifications require the same surgical cure as hypercalcemic PHPT.
- Post-operative care in the first days and months, which can lead to serious complications.

I don't doubt you will understand our concerns when you read our members experiences. The current guideline provides a tool to back up poor treatment decisions. It reinforces the idea that patients have no entitlement to a surgical cure (parathyroidectomy) until they have end-organ damage such as kidney stones or osteoporosis, unless they have calcium greater than 2.85mmol/L.

The reality is that many people with much lower levels over long periods of time, are more likely to have kidney stones and osteoporosis, but they will be told incorrectly their calcium levels are not high enough to cause them. Economically, you will appreciate the effect these ideas have on NHS resources. There are too many endocrinologists employed by each NHS Trust, often with too few or even none of them having up to date knowledge of all classifications of PHPT.

They keep patients on their recall lists year upon year when they could be discharged after a successful parathyroidectomy. This can impact other departments such as urology, A&E, rheumatology, haematology, physiotherapy, fracture, bone and pain clinics.

We see an opportunity for the NHS to save a great deal of money by reducing the number of endocrinologists per hospital who are not effectively helping patients. We recommend this solution to save you money and also to help patients. Each NHS Trust should have a specifically trained PHPT endocrinologist to refer patients to. If patients can learn enough to be up to date with primary hyperparathyroidism in all classifications, endocrinologists can easily be brought up to speed. We have a website that can help with this process; **Hyperparathyroiduk.com**.

We are in contact with several surgeons who fully recognise, and operate on patients with all classifications of PHPT, but there are not enough of them. I highly recommend Mr Shad Khan at Oxford University Hospitals; Shahab.khan@ouh.nhs.uk if you would like to discuss the current situation regarding PHPT with him. Please do look at the some of his case stories on our website.

Kind regards

Sallie Powell
Founder/CEO Hyperparathyroid UK
Hyperparathyroiduk.com

Event Letter to Amanda Howe from Hyperparathyroid UK

Monday 15 March 2021
Our Ref: SJP/AH-RCGP/15-03-21

Dear Amanda Howe

RE: Action needed by RCGP for recognition and treatment of Primary Hyperparathyroidism (PHPT)

I am writing to you as the CEO of Hyperparathyroid UK, founded in September 2014, to ask you to read this letter and others being sent to you today from some of our members. We have three issues to raise;

- Very poor understanding of Primary Hyperparathyroidism symptoms, leading to misinformation from many GPs to patients about calcium levels and symptoms of PHPT.
- PHPT misdiagnosed as fibromyalgia/CFS/ menopause, causes delays in referrals to endocrine consultants which often amounts to decades for some patients.
- Poor understanding of blood tests required to test for/rule out PHPT and understanding the results.

We accept that General Practitioners are not experts on conditions, but we find it unacceptable that so many GPs have such a poor understanding of PHPT, that it is causing extreme delays in referrals which not only causes harm to patients but also impacts economically on the number of GP consultations required by them, as well as impacting many departments in secondary care such as rheumatology, A&E, Urology, haematology, physiotherapy, fracture, bone and pain clinics.

In 2016 we wrote to Sir Bruce Keogh to ask him to initiate the process of commissioning NICE guidelines for PHPT. We were grateful he obliged. Professor Mark Baker wrote to tell me RCGP had commissioned them and suggested we become registered stakeholders. Sadly, the guideline committee failed to consider the comments and evidence our members (NHS patients) submitted during the public consultations. The result of those omissions contribute to devastating impacts on patients' health, which can result in A&E admissions. It also impacts them socially, with many forced to withdraw from society. The important information they omitted;

- Information relating to two classifications of PHPT; normocalcemic PHPT and normohormonal PHPT. Both classifications require the same surgical cure as hypercalcemic PHPT.
- Post-operative care in the first days and months, which can lead to serious complications.

We need our GPs to recognise all classifications of PHPT, to understand the suppressive relationship between calcium and parathyroid hormone in order to understand the above classifications, and to recognise that calcium, PTH (specified to be tested in EDTA vials), vitamin D and magnesium are all crucial starting points for tests. Patients need their doctors to know the following;

- Low vitamin D does not rule out Primary HPT if calcium falls within the normal range. It may indicate Secondary HPT if calcium is below range with an elevated or high normal PTH
- Calcium and PTH both falling within the normal range does not exclude PHPT. Where they fall in the range is crucial to diagnosis. A patient with a calcium level of 2.58mmol/L without a suppressed PTH could be very unwell, developing kidney stones or bone density loss. The body may well be excreting calcium via the kidneys. A 24hr urine sample must be requested in symptomatic patients in these cases.
- It is impossible to rule out PHPT by testing calcium alone, a concept believed by too many doctors. This understanding must be eradicated with some urgency.
- Patients discharged to their primary care doctors after their parathyroidectomy are faced with GPs who have no idea how to help them. It is crucial GPs understand bone remineralisation post parathyroidectomy, and its effect on calcium, vitamin D and magnesium. This understanding can prevent many A&E admissions for patients experiencing low calcium levels. Understanding how vitamin D and magnesium work with remineralisation and calcium absorption is vital.

We are able to help all the patients before or after surgery, who find our support group and/or our website. We are very concerned for patients who do not find us. If patients can learn enough to be up to date with PHPT, primary care doctors can easily be brought up to speed. Please do refer your GPs to our website to help them to learn how to help their patients; hyperparathyroiduk.com

We believe the NICE guideline for PHPT; (https://www.nice.org.uk/guidance/NG132) let down patients and their GPs and also RCGP who commissioned them. They do not help your doctors to help their patients. We are writing to Sir Simon Stevens and the NHS CEO's in Wales, and Scotland, as well as the Ministers for Health in Ireland and Northern Ireland today. The problem of misdiagnosis and poor treatment recommendations is far reaching around the UK. We would very much appreciate your assistance with all of the above, and your help to commission an urgently needed update to the NICE guidelines.

Kind regards

Sallie Powell
Founder/CEO of Hyperparathyroid UK
Hyperparathyroiduk.com

Alyson Blythe

Dear Simon and Amanda,

I was born and raised in London but I now live in the USA (near Washington DC). I suffered with Normohormonal Parathyroid disease for thirteen years. During this time I had numerous trips to the A&E both in the US and in England as I lived in both countries for a period of this time.

My symptoms were wide ranging but my gastro issues and heart palpitations were the ones that sent me to A&E. Finally in 2018 I went in desperation to John's Hopkins Hospital in Baltimore Maryland and my "slightly elevated Calcium" was followed up on with a blood test for PTH which came back in the normal range. Fortunately I paid attention and although the diagnosis was dismissed, I decided to investigate Primary Hyperparathyroidism, as after a cursory google, I felt like I was reading about my symptoms. Four days later I attended their After Care Clinic and insisted on being tested again. Again they dismissed the diagnosis of PHPT. At this point, I was convinced I had the disease and submitted my bloodwork to The Norman Parathyroid Clinic in Tampa, Florida. I simultaneously downloaded their App "Calcium Pro" and entered my blood results only to find that the result was 'highly likely' I had the disease. (That App won an award in 2024 as the Medical App of the year award). Just imagine how I felt after years of suffering, to see that confirmation.

No doctor in all of those A&E visits paid any attention to my slightly high calcium. We have the same problem here in the USA.

Three weeks after my discovery I had one gland removed that when probed was excreting 877 units of parathyroid hormone in a normally accepted range of 30-60.

No wonder I felt like I was dying.

I know you have many emails and letters so I won't list all of my symptoms over the years of suffering, and will cut my story short here, but suffice to say that something needs to be done about this life robbing disease. No one knows this more than us, the short and long term sufferers. It's a torturous illness and I have a lot of bitterness about lost years so it still haunts me.

Please listen to us; - and act.

My GP here in the USA has said that one day we will write a paper together. She learned so much from me about this illness and has tested and sent 10 other patients for Parathyroidectomies based on her learning from me. Knowledgeable physicians are lifesavers! I'm here in Sallie's group to help other sufferers. In my research I found this Facebook support group and learned about my illness.

Without it, I don't know where, or if I would still be here today,

Thank you for taking the time to read this.

Alyson Blythe

Allison Tait

Our Ref: SJP/AH-RCGP/15-03-21
15TH March 2021

Dear Amanda Howe

RE: Action needed by NHS England for recognition and treatment of Hyperparathyroidism

I am writing to you as a member of Hyperparathyroid UK.

My story may be a little different to most, but it just goes to show that there are very few doctors and endocrinologists out there with enough background knowledge or even awareness of Hyperparathyroidism.

In January 2017 my Hyperparathyroidism was picked up after having a routine blood test by my GP, who immediately made me an appointment with an endocrinologist while I was sat in her surgery.

In April 2017 I attended hospital for the appointment with an endocrinologist who looked at my blood results and diagnosed me with Primary Hyperparathyroidism. He went on to explain to me that the only cure for this disease was surgery. At first I was very reluctant for surgery to take place as, at that time. I simply did not have any symptoms. However, within the space of a few months I became quite ill with fatigue and bone pain mainly, but the list goes on. I telephoned my endocrinologist who immediately put me forward for surgery.

I met with the surgeon in November 2017 and in January 2018 I had a successful parathyroidectomy.

As not many people had heard of this disease I was lucky to find the group Hyperparathyroid UK to which Sallie and all of the members were an amazing source of morale support.
Of course, most of the stories are not like mine, as most of the members have had to fight for surgery, when this should not be the

case, and my story proves this. Ideally, there should be more general awareness of this debilitating illness within the medical profession.

Kind Regards

Mrs Allison Tait

Ange Tegg

Dear Sir Simon Stevens,

I write in support of letter reference SJP/SS-CEO NHS/15-03-21 to highlight the ongoing struggles I am experiencing with hyperparathyroidism, and to hopefully raise awareness of not only the devastating effect it can have on people's health and lives but also to highlight the wasted NHS money, time and resources, due to late diagnosis and delayed treatment of this illness.

Although it was only in spring of last year (2020) that I was diagnosed as having hyperparathyroidism, my symptoms began seven years ago. I first went to see my GP about extreme fatigue and exhaustion, a year after my second daughter was born in 2013. I noticed a considerable difference in my energy levels and how much my bones ached in comparison to what I experienced after the birth of my first child; some days, my hands and arms ached so much, I could barely lift her and I struggled so badly with fatigue and aches, that short walks seemed impossible. This was alien to me - after the birth of my first child, I found my fitness came back quickly and I was easily running 3-5k a day; now I was struggling to walk for five minutes.

I was informed by my GP that this was normal, that I was exhausted with two young children, and that I needed to prioritise sleep and nutrition. A few months later, now 2014, I started to have serious stomach pains, cramps, swelling, tenderness in my stomach when I ate, and the fatigue was now dominating my life. I visited the doctor three times due to pain in my bones, fatigue and stomach issues. I was told it was all stress-related due to working and being a mum. This seemed very strange to me - I didn't feel stressed in the slightest, I loved my part time job and I loved being a mum. I had a brilliant support network around me.

The doctor had asked me "are you really doing everything you can to look after yourself?" Yes. I was. I left feeling completely embarrassed and like I had to try harder to exercise, eat healthily and sleep more. And I did. I cut my working hours down to one and a half days a week and asked for more help and support from grandparents and my husband, so that I could rest. Nothing made a difference. I accepted that this was all part of being a mum to two at age 33 and that exhaustion and pain were just normal for my circumstances.

In 2016 I started to experience pain in the left hand side of my neck, ear and jaw. After several GP appointments I was referred to ENT at West Suffolk Hospital for an endoscopy, which showed nothing in my throat. The doctors decided to remove my tonsils in 2017 to see if this was causing the pain. However, there was no improvement after this and although I returned to ENT after the tonsillectomy, twice with the same pain and fatigue, I was told the pain was most likely muscular and I would need physiotherapy, and that the tonsillectomy had been unnecessary.

I had the most uncomfortable appointment with a doctor who made me feel awful for making a fuss and having a procedure that didn't need doing. I felt personally responsible for wasting NHS time and money and went home to crack on with the pain and fatigue, again trying to convince myself that I just had to learn to live with this and I was obviously making a fuss. In 2018, sick of feeling fatigued, in pain and not listened to, I decided to start running again, something I had always enjoyed and found easy previous to 2013. I believed if I could get my fitness back on track all of the other symptoms would subside. After two weeks of running, I was back at the doctors with severe hip, knee, ankle and back pain and swelling in my knees and ankles - my back had literally 'gone' and I was unable to walk for a few days. I was referred to physiotherapy, where after several appointments I was referred for an x-ray on my lower back, which showed deterioration of my lower vertebrae. I was told to stop running but keep up with walking, swimming, cycling, and yoga. Again, I was told that this was just part of getting older (I was 39 at this stage and now starting to feel depressed that my body was in this much pain and my energy levels depleted).

Between 2018 and 2020 I became unbelievably fatigued, having to take afternoon naps, no longer being able to exercise with my young children, unable to enjoy social events because I just needed to be in bed so early. Often my husband would take the children out for family days and I would stay home in bed, resting and sleeping. The pain in my neck had become worse and I was sent for an MRI scan which didn't show anything. I began to believe that this was what being 40 was like and I had to accept it.

In 2019, I returned to my GP with pain in my neck and complete burn out. I was told I had to accept the pain in my neck as it was most likely scar tissue from the tonsillectomy and I would have it for some time. I was sent for bloods which showed raised calcium. The GP told me to be aware I may develop kidney stones. No further tests were done. I left feeling like something else was wrong with me and I honestly could not believe this was my health and my life aged forty.

In January of 2020, I had appendicitis and had my appendix removed. The biopsy showed abnormalities and I was referred for a colonoscopy. I am still unsure whether these were related but have since found from research that raised calcium plays havoc with other organs and causes all manner of stomach problems. In discussions with my GP and endocrinologist, it has been suggested that PHPT may have contributed, if not caused this.

In spring 2020, I had severe pain in my lower left back. I saw a different GP who sent me for bloods. I was called back the same day to be told he suspected it was kidney stones and that I had an illness called primary hyperparathyroidism. As he sat in front of me explaining the symptoms, I couldn't help but cry, not that I was being told I had this awful illness, but out of sheer relief that everything he was describing accounted for the symptoms I had been experiencing since at least 2013.

I was sent for nuclear imaging and ultrasound scans on my neck and finally, an 11mm lesion was found on the left of my neck and a 3mm adenoma was found on the right of my neck. Hyperparathyroidism was confirmed, and again, I was so relieved to know that I had not been imagining the pain in my neck. I was excited that this was finally getting sorted. I have since found out that hyperparathyroidism can cause miscarriage; I experienced several miscarriages and an ectopic pregnancy between 2008 and 2013 and now wonder if my PHPT goes back further than 2013.

The mental health struggles that many of us experience due to brain fog, anxiety and forgetfulness due to raised calcium levels, are also concerning, but this is exacerbated by the fact diagnosis takes so long that many patients report experiencing depression and frustration at being repeatedly told there is nothing wrong with them when we know that there is. The feeling of not being heard, of being patronised, of being contradicted and undermined is simply dreadful and I can tell you first hand that eight years to get a diagnosis is too long for a young woman (or anyone) desperate to live a full and rich life with her children and family.

My career in teaching has been seriously hampered by having to decrease my hours due to exhaustion and again the impact this has had on me mentally has caused a great deal of distress. Since being diagnosed with HPT last year, I have been on a waiting list for an operation but due to Covid-19 this has been pushed back. I have had two trips to the GP recently with numbness down my left arm, in the left of my face, swollen left armpit, pains in my bones, chest pains, ECG and more bloods. I experience kidney stone pain almost every day but until I have my operation nothing can be done about my kidney stones or deep bone pain, which they believe is osteoporosis, caused by hyperparathyroidism. The plethora of symptoms I am developing is increasing as I wait for an operation that I desperately need.

I am writing this letter today, in the hope that I can raise awareness about the importance of early diagnosis, not only for the benefit of people who suffer from this terrible illness but also due to the wasted money, time and resources for the NHS. An early blood test of my PTH and calcium with early diagnosis and treatment would have avoided eight years of wasted appointments, blood tests, operations, physiotherapy appointments, medication, scans and hospital stays. This illness has ruined my life and taken years away from me that I should have been enjoying with my family. Eight years for a diagnosis has no doubt drained unnecessary NHS resources and this all could have been avoided with early diagnosis and treatment. I hope that by writing this letter, people in the future will not have to endure the pain, delays, frustration, and deterioration in their health, that so many of us are living with and I hope that the wasted NHS funds will be used more effectively elsewhere. Thank you for taking the time to read this.

Regards

Ange Tegg

Anita Kittle

Ref SJP/SS-CEO NHS/15-03-21

Dear Sir Simon Stevens,

Further to Sallie Powell's letter as above, regarding primary hyperparathyroidism, I am writing to you about my experience with this awful disease.

I started noticing my symptoms in November 2019. I saw my GP who prescribed an antidepressant and migraine melts. I had lost my Mum in August 2019 so at the time my GP understandably, put my symptoms down to grief. I was having daily headaches, regular migraines, fatigue; generally no 'get up and go'. I had gone from walking regularly to sleeping a lot.

My symptoms continued and I revisited my GP in February 2020 where bloods were requested. These indicated low vitamin D, low calcium and high PTH. I was referred to an endocrinologist (private healthcare) who prescribed six weeks of high dose vitamin D3. Repeat bloods were done and I had high PTH, normal calcium, normal vitamin D. I was told to have repeat bloods in three to six months, and was diagnosed with primary hyperparathyroidism.

Unfortunately in August 2020, I had to visit Colchester A&E with horrific pain and vomiting. I had many kidney stones (one known cause of primary hyperparathyroidism). I was instructed to see my endocrinologist again as soon as possible.

My GP kindly referred me to an urologist for my kidney stone problem privately and I had two operations in September and November 2020 to remove stones from both kidneys. These were identified as calcium oxalate stones. Unfortunately from December 2020 to date I have had six UTI's and eight prescriptions for antibiotics. I have recently found out that another calcium stone (8mm) has grown.

I met with my endocrinologist who ordered an ultrasound (a positive adenoma was seen) and a nuclear scan (this did not highlight anything) and a 24hr urine collection (acceptable calcium levels) all under my private healthcare.

I met again with my endocrinologist to discuss next steps, feeling positive that we had found the problem. Unfortunately he would not refer me to a surgeon even though I had kidney stones and a positive scan. Apparently I had to have osteoporosis to get to see a surgeon. My endocrinologist suggested a dexa scan which came back as above average levels. Due to the bone scan being normal, my endocrinologist said there was nothing else he could do and to repeat bloods in nine to twelve months. I was exhausted.

My GP and urologist were now getting frustrated as they did not want me to go through the kidney stone pain again and the affect it can have on the kidneys.

I decided to get a second opinion, a surgeon this time privately. Again I was palmed off and it was suggested that I saw a rheumatologist… All because I had normal calcium.

Fortunately, I found an amazing parathyroid support group on Facebook run by Sallie Powell and her team. I was overwhelmed by their support and advice. I could not believe how many others are/were suffering with normal calcium levels and being put to the side just like me.

It was recommended that I got in touch with Mr Shahab Khan at Oxford University Hospitals who could look at my bloods and scans. My very cooperative GP, Mr Imran Ramjan at Winstree Medical Practice, Colchester, Essex, kindly referred me to him (privately) as he was just as concerned and frustrated as me. I am so glad I got referred to Mr Khan. What an asset to the NHS you have! He looked at all the information and was surprised I had not been offered surgery, especially as I had kidney stones, positive scan and high PTH.

I was fortunate enough to have my parathyroidectomy on 23 January 2021 (I chose to do this privately). Mr Khan found that I had parathyroid hyperplasia. All four glands were abnormal. Three were removed and one was left. The removed glands were 12mm, 11mm and 9mm in size. PTH blood results have indicated a cure which is amazing. I do not know how long my glands were abnormal

Can I please ask that the NICE guidelines for primary hyperparathyroidism dated 23 May 2019 are reviewed? So many patients are suffering which in turn is costing the NHS even more money for other tests, treatments and operations, which puts pressure on other departments. Some of us have had to go private as we have felt so unwell and cannot live our lives. I have been unable to work but hopefully in a few months I will feel better and can start looking.

If you have had the chance to read my story, thank you for your time, especially during a pandemic.

I am forever grateful to Mr Khan and my GP.

I also want to thank A&E Colchester and the radiology department.

The NHS is truly a wonderful asset to this country and I would like to extend a huge thank you to all employees and volunteers. Well done.

Yours sincerely,

Anita Kittle

Anita Reilly

Dear Simon

It is with sad news I have to write this, but please, please hear my story.

I was diagnosed with primary hyperparathyroidism, and left as a 'watch and wait' case for nine years.

Endocrinologists and doctors didn't think my calcium levels were 'that' elevated. They ranged from 2.48 - 2.78mmol/L, depending on when they were done and if done correctly!

Sadly, I'm a wreck these days with constant hospital appointments for all the issue I now have. Two years ago I went privately to a surgeon who gave me a scan and found one parathyroid adenoma! I had a parathyroidectomy and they found three adenomas!

All those hospital appointments wasted because nobody really knew what to look for, and all that money wasted with medications and scans and years of my life!

I spent nine years thinking I was going mad; not nice. My home life, work and social life all suffered because nobody listens and I felt like a whingey old bag. I was 50 and felt 80.

Please get this awful disease recognised and the levels of calcium requiring surgery changed. A parathyroidectomy is the only answer and these archaic ways must stop. We need your help now.

Thank you for your time.

Anita Reilly

Anna Gibbs

Dear Sir

I write in support of letter reference SJP/SS-CEONHS/15-03-21 to share my experience of primary hyperparathyroidism.

I am one of the lucky ones who found Sallie's Facebook support group at the start of my diagnosis. Through the group I was able to access the specialised help I required.

I have had several years of increasing bone and joint pain which was diagnosed as arthritis. I was therefore prescribed a variety of painkillers culminating in Tramadol. I also suffered from high blood pressure, gastric reflux, ectopy, depression, insomnia, fatigue, anxiety and brain fog.

I visited a locum GP who actually listened to me and ordered a set of blood tests which I have annually. The blood tests in February 2020, for the first time ever included a calcium check, which showed high calcium. My usual GP then repeated the tests and added PTH and vitamin D. These showed the calcium had slightly decreased but the PTH levels were high. I had an appointment with yet another GP who printed off some information on hyperparathyroidism and told me that as I was over fifty, there was nothing more to be done. Although I was sixty seven at the time, I refused to accept there was no cure for me, and luckily found the Facebook support group.

At my request, blood tests were repeated in August. My GP was then willing to refer me to an endocrinologist but he didn't think I would be suitable for surgery. Again I turned to the group and through it, I found Mr Shad Khan, a surgeon at the Churchill Hospital in Oxford. My GP then agreed to refer me there.

Following an initial consultation in September, I had surgery in November. Three large glands were removed. Just by looking at my blood results, Mr Khan had no doubt that surgery was necessary. The difference in my mood is dramatic and many of my other symptoms are reduced. As it can take up to year for levels to stabilise I feel very hopeful.

I am one of the lucky ones because a young locum GP saw a pattern to my symptoms. I am lucky in that I am able to question being written off because of my age. I am lucky because I found the PHPT support group. I am lucky that Mr Khan is willing to engage with patient support groups. Sadly the majority of sufferers are not as lucky. The NHS should not rely on luck.

- The large scale misdiagnosis of PHPT due to lack of education needs to stop.
- NICE guidelines need updating.
- Poor knowledge of PHPT, leading to 'a watch and wait' approach compared to parathyroidectomy is causing the NHS to waste resources as well as ruining many lives.

I hope you will take on board the experiences of people suffering from this condition and act accordingly.

Yours sincerely

Anna Gibbs

Anne McDonald

Dear Mr Stevens

<u>I write in support of letter SJP/SS-CEO NHS/15-03-21.</u>

I am a sixty seven year old lady. I was diagnosed with primary hyperparathyroidism in 2015. In January 2021 I finally had a parathyroidectomy; a 15mm adenoma was removed by Mr Shad Khan at Oxford University Hospitals.

During the previous six years, I attended many hospital appointments at Royal University Hospital, Bath. I was seen by at least five different endocrinologists, was misdiagnosed, and underwent at least six different scans. In contrast, I approached Mr Khan in November 2020, and was cured by January 2021!

Because of hesitation or misguided training, my quality of life has been severely affected. During these 'wait and see' years, I have developed osteoporosis and chronic kidney disease. My other symptoms of this horrible disease included terrible mood swings, anxiety and exhaustion which were not taken seriously by the so called experts on this disease.

Sadly, my forty four year marriage did not survive, and I blame my symptoms for this. I hope you will look at ways to avoid my experience happening to future patients of primary hyperparathyroidism.

Yours sincerely

Ann McDonald

Barbara Harding

Hyperparathyroid UK Ref: SJP/SS-CEO NHS/15-03-21

Dear Sir Simon Stevens

I am writing in support of the letter sent to you by Sallie Powell of the group Hyperparathyroid UK - Action4Change as referenced above.

Currently I have a diagnosis of Primary Hyperparathyroidism and Osteoporosis and I am on the waiting list for a 'bilateral neck exploration' surgery. Of course due to the current pandemic situation I do not know when that might happen however I have been told that it is likely to be up to a one year wait.

I am 72 years old and have had Fibromyalgia for many years, my GP's in UK never gave a proper diagnosis or support but when we lived in Austria for a few years I was diagnosed and some help provided. However in 2009 I began to feel some different symptoms and went to my GP. I was referred to a rheumatologist and after blood testing was told my calcium levels were high but that a parathyroid hormone blood test was ok. With no more explanation I was told it must be still Fibromyalgia.

In 2016 I felt sufficiently bad to have a private blood test looking for answers. They said my vitamin D was low and that I should take supplements but that was all. Their figures showed that my calcium was quite high but this was not mentioned in the report. The vitamin D did not seem to help my symptoms.

Late 2019 I began to have heart palpitations which were quite worrying. I thought maybe it was anxiety after a family crisis a few months earlier. The GP sent me to A&E where they said it was not a heart attack but that my calcium was high and that I should be checked for parathyroid issues. This was when I first started to look on the internet, and began to realise that a lot of the hyperparathyroid symptoms fitted with what I had been going through.

Throughout 2020 I had tests, scans and remote consultations and ended up with a diagnosis and referral to a surgeon. I can't complain at all about the process last year especially given all the difficulties for the NHS. My results fitted the NICE guidelines so I am now waiting to go ahead and gradually feeling worse all the time. I have manage to learn which supplements will help from the Facebook site for group Hyperparathyroid UK - Action4Change and I am very grateful to them for their help and knowledge.

This is a debilitating illness and I appreciate that people present with it in many different ways. I also appreciate that the medical profession is still coming to grips with the best (and most cost effective) way of helping those of us suffering with it. My experience so far is that Sallie Powell and her team have an excellent understanding of what is needed to help everyone to move forward and hope that you will be able to use her input constructively for the future.

Kind Regards

Barbara Harding

Carol

Our Ref: SJP/AH-RCGP/15-03-21
Monday 15 March 2021

Dear Sir Simon Stevens

RE: Action needed by RCGP for recognition and treatment of Primary Hyperparathyroidism.

I am writing to you in support of the letter sent to you by Sallie Powell, founder/CEO of Hyperparathyroid UK. I joined this patient support group following a diagnosis of primary hyperparathyroidism (PHPT) last year.

I was fortunate to have a diligent GP who suspected PHPT following a raised blood calcium result. He commented at that time that many GP colleagues would probably not investigate further as it was only 'slightly raised'. I was also fortunate to be referred to an endocrinologist who had no hesitation in confirming a diagnosis of PHPT.

I am aware that sadly many patients elsewhere in the country have not experienced my prompt diagnosis. Members of Hyperparathyroid UK with similar blood results and symptoms to my own, have described very poor experiences as they struggle to obtain a correct diagnosis and treatment. I have read many accounts from patients who have been left to suffer the debilitating effects of this condition for several years due to a delayed diagnosis, a 'watch and wait' approach, or even misdiagnosis. Long-term harm, including osteoporosis, kidney stones, and other end-organ damage become more likely the longer PHPT is left untreated.

The Covid pandemic has of course, delayed elective surgeries across the UK. I am coping with many symptoms as well as osteoporosis while waiting for curative surgery a year after my diagnosis. This week I have been told I face 'a very long wait' for surgery under the NHS because my blood levels do not warrant an urgent operation. I do not have private health insurance – I am a great supporter of the

NHS and worked for the NHS for almost twenty five years. However, I have made the decision to pay for private surgery rather than suffer further deterioration to my physical and mental health.

I am thankful that I have not been subjected to a 'watch and wait' approach by my GP or endocrinologist, and recognise, that in normal times, I probably would be having surgery under the NHS within a reasonable timescale.

The costs to NHS England both in primary and secondary care, must be greater when diagnosis and curative surgery are delayed. With consistent and improved standards of treatment of PHPT across the NHS, I believe savings could be achieved and patients' health improved.

Yours sincerely

Carol

Charulata Shah

Dear Sir Simon Stevens/Professor Amanda Howe

RE: Action needed by NHS England for recognition and treatment of Hyperparathyroidism.

I am writing to you as a member of the Facebook Group. Hyperparathyroid UK – Action4Change, established by Sallie Powell in 2014 and which has provided immeasurable support to hundreds of patients of the endocrine condition Hyperparathyroidism, including myself. As a Group, we have three issues to raise:

The scale of misdiagnosis and misinformation to patients with primary hyperparathyroidism (PHPT), by many consultants, including endocrinologists, throughout the NHS, which causes prolonged treatment delays and can cause harm. We recognise the root is poor education at many levels throughout the NHS.

- We request an immediate update to NICE guideline for PHPT; https://www.nice.org.uk/guidance/NG132 to help many patients excluded by them, based on calcium levels. We consider them to be a failure and that they appear to have been engineered to steer patients away from the NHS, and towards private care with their prohibitive surgical restrictions.
- Immense waste of NHS resources led by poor knowledge of PHPT. To quote Mr Shad Khan, Consultant Surgeon at Oxford University Hospitals; 'Studies looking at the cost effectiveness of parathyroidectomy compared to medical management show that surgery is far superior economically overall; https://www.surgjournal.com/article/S0039-6060(16)30493-7/fulltext.

In 2016 the Group wrote to Sir Bruce Keogh to ask him to initiate the process of commissioning NICE guidelines for PHPT. We were grateful he obliged. We became registered stakeholders. Sadly, the guideline committee failed to consider the comments and evidence, we as NHS patients submitted during the public consultations. The result of those omissions contribute to devastating impacts on patients, which can result in A&E admissions. The important information they omitted;

- Information relating to two classifications of PHPT; normocalcaemic PHPT and normohormonal PHPT. Both classifications require the same surgical cure as hypercalcaemic PHPT.
- Post-operative care in the first days and months, which can lead to serious complications.

Due to the existing NICE guideline, endocrinologists in the UK failed to diagnose me with Normocalcaemic Hyperparathyroidism between 2016 and 2019. No NHS or Private consultant was willing to take me seriously as I struggled with numerous symptoms and my quality of life deteriorated because my blood test results did not fit the picture of a 'typical' hyperparathyroid patent.

I then decided to advocate for myself rather than rely on the UK health system and sought help from a notable US specialist, Mr Babak Larian MD based in Los Angeles, USA. I was one of the fortunate ones because using my personal savings and financial help from my family, I was able to travel to the US in May 2019 to have a parathyroidectomy and have three out of my four glands removed due to hyperplasia (enlarged glands giving rise to high parathyroid hormone levels) in a successful surgery. However, it cost me nearly **£16,000** to do this due to the lack of expertise in the NHS.

I should NEVER have had to resort to this, had the NICE guideline recognised Normocalcaemic Hyperparathyroidism, but sheer desperation drove me to it. If you've ever been unwell for a long period of time (and I hope you haven't or never are) then you would understand the frustration of repeatedly being told there is nothing wrong with you. The sheer lack of awareness of this condition across consultants, so-called specialists etc. in the UK is embarrassing and quite frankly diabolical.

I find it completely illogical that Calcium, Vitamin D and Parathyroid Hormone (PTH) are not routinely tested as a triad rather than individually. The vast waste of expense that would be removed by this one simple process would make a huge difference. Prior to surgery, I was diagnosed with osteopenia, the precursor to osteoporosis at the age of 46. Osteopenia is reversible if caused by Hyperparathyroidism, provided a patient has timely surgery to cure the problem. My osteopenia has already improved since surgery

This is one condition where surgery actually provides patients with a permanent cure to the condition. But the hurdles a patient has to go through via the NHS due to various factors like a lack of awareness, an ill-informed NICE guideline, a skewed logic, that reflects a reluctance to cure but a willingness to treat and medically manage, etc. makes it virtually impossible to be treated. There are hundreds of actual and potential patients in the Group who are there to help guide and advise each other based on our experiences and accumulated knowledge. We are not medically trained and we do not claim to be, but we fill a huge gap of providing support to those who are suffering, and don't know what to do or have lost hope of ever regaining their health back.

I don't doubt you will understand our concerns when you read our Group members' experiences. The current guideline provides a tool to back up poor treatment decisions. It reinforces the idea that patients have no entitlement to a surgical cure (parathyroidectomy) until they have end-organ damage such as kidney stones or osteoporosis, unless they have calcium greater than 2.85mmol/L. The reality is that many people with much lower levels over long periods of time are more likely to have kidney stones and osteoporosis, but they will be told incorrectly their calcium levels are not high enough to cause them. Economically you will appreciate the effect these ideas have on NHS resources. There are too many endocrinologists employed by each NHS Trust, often with too few or even none of them having up to date knowledge of all classifications of PHPT. They keep patients on their recall lists year upon year when they could be discharged after a successful parathyroidectomy. We see an opportunity for the NHS to save a great deal of money by reducing the number of endocrinologists per hospital, who are not effectively helping patients. This can impact other departments such as urology, A&E, rheumatology, haematology, physiotherapy, fracture, bone and pain clinics. We can recommend some solutions to save you money and to help patients;

- Each NHS Trust has a specifically trained PHPT endocrinologist to refer patients to. If patients can learn enough to be up to date with PHPT, endocrinologists can easily be brought up to speed. We believe efficient change can greatly reduce the number of endocrinologists required.

- Our Group has a website that can help with this process; Hyperparathyroiduk.com

I look forward to hearing from you.

Kind regards

Ms Charulata Shah

Chris Walton 1

Dear Amanda

Please find attached a letter I have sent to Simon Stevens today.

There is a real opportunity within General Practice for GPs to spot hyperparathyroidism early and implement solutions. Take sick patients with often "woolly" symptoms, out of primary and secondary investigations and straight to more cost effective surgery.

Hyperparathyroidism is not a condition that goes away and the blood results do not need a 'wait and see' policy - by which time damage can have been done to a patient. My GP has given me great care - apart from with regard to this condition. That suggests that it's the absence of good guidelines for general practice that is at the root cause of the delays in giving the right care to patients. Had the guidelines been clearer I would have been diagnosed sooner, more cost effectively, and would have been on the road to recovery by now.

I hope my letter and email makes sense and that you can lend your support to our request for better care for people with hyperparathyroidism

Kind regards

Christine Walton

Dear Sir Simon Stevens,

I am writing in support of the letter you will have received from Sallie Powell, Founder/CEO of Hyperparathyroid UK.

Although a common endocrine condition, primary hyperparathyroidism is poorly recognised in the NHS, in both primary and secondary care. As a result, patients often wait years for the right diagnosis, and the symptoms long term are life shortening - kidney problems, osteoporosis and cardiac disease. Along this path symptoms are debilitating and wide ranging. Many people have to give up work, have poor life experiences etc. GPs are not fully aware of the condition and as a result persevere with a range of unnecessary misdirected investigations and referrals, which cost the NHS an immense amount, and clog up the service with patients who do not need to be there. It can take years for the right diagnosis and by that time many patients are left with irreversible damage. Most of these health problems and costs could be avoided.

Here is my own experience – you will forgive lapses of date and timings, brain fog is a typical symptom.

I was a freelance IT project manager, who first had hip replacements and a revision, as one had been put in wrongly. This took up the first three years of my 50s. I then passed out and was told incorrectly by a neurologist that I had 24/7 migraine. At one of many neck and brain scans I overheard the radiographers' state that I had C5/6 problems. I was able to pick this up with another hospital – the Royal Orthopaedic Hospital in Birmingham, who correctly reviewed and diagnosed C5/6 problems and I had ACDF surgery.

This resolved some of my problems, however I still had extreme fatigue, brain fog, hand and arm pain and heaviness, which prevented me from working.

My GP referred me back to another neurologist. I went for more brain scans and was told that I did not have MS, Parkinson's or

Motor Neurone Disease and that he was at a loss. He referred me back to the orthopaedic team at the Royal Orthopaedic Hospital and suggested a second set of nerve conductive studies and also blood tests. The GP did the tests, reviewed the test results and arranged for me to be checked for a very unusual condition - Familial Hypocalciuric Hypercalcemia. She did not look at a differential diagnosis of primary hyperparathyroidism (PHPT), which is far more common. Fortunately her request to check my results landed with an excellent endocrinologist who understood PHPT. He reviewed the results, and said I had biochemical PHPT. I arranged to see this endocrinologist privately so that I could get some better understanding and support. It took years to get to this point. It should have taken weeks.

By good fortune a friend of mine recommended the Hyperparathyroid UK site. This site has been a lifeline to many people with the condition. It has given guidance on how to take control of our situations. As a result of the sites guidance, I looked through my previous blood tests and provided them to the private endocrinologist. I have since had follow up through the NHS and I am now waiting for a parathyroidectomy. In the meantime, I have brain fog, immense fatigue, memory loss, heavy hands and arms, and nerve pain. The team at the Royal Orthopaedic Hospital who are still looking into my hand and arm pain, weakness and pain are not prepared to take action, until I have had my parathyroid surgery, as my symptoms may be related to the PHPT, not an orthopaedic problem. So even though I am on the right track there is still some way to go. My C5/6 surgery was in October 2017 and my hyperparathyroidism diagnosis was summer of 2020. Three lost years.

Put simply I have lost really valuable working years – I was at the top of my game. I have lost irreplaceable time with family and friends – needing to rest and sleep and being in immense pain, instead of enjoying the active outdoors that was at the centre of my life. I skied, rock climbed, rambled, sailed and wind surfed, and cycled. I can't do any of these anymore.

I have clogged up my surgery with appointments and my GP has spent an arm and a leg trying to get me diagnosed, when all he had to do was look at the calcium and vitamin D results, my symptoms, and then run a combined calcium, vitamin D and parathyroid hormone blood test. This would have identified the condition years before, and my life would have been very different. Instead my GP has suggested that I may have ME, or fibromyalgia and/or depression, suggested as the root cause of my symptoms. GPs need support and education in spotting and dealing with this condition.

When I have ended up being referred to a specialist, then when that person ran out of ideas, then I was referred for further secondary investigations in a different specialism. I can only wonder at how many other people with this condition bounce around the NHS primary and secondary sectors for years. The unlucky ones develop very serious conditions, before they are diagnosed.

This letter is personal and about my own experiences. I think they are not that different for many other people who have hyperparathyroidism. We need diagnosis and treatment quickly to get us back to a normal life. The diagnosis and treatment path are simple and relatively cheap, compared to the long term damage and high cost to the NHS, of incorrectly diagnosing patients, who then need expensive interventions and may have irreversible damage.

Yours sincerely

Christine Walton

Copied by email to

Amanda Howe

President of the Royal College of General Practitioners

Claire Friend

Our Ref SJP/SS-CEO NHS/15-03-21

RE: Action needed by NHS England for recognition and treatment of Hyperparathyroidism

I am writing to you as a member of the action group Hyperparathyroid UK.

I am also a sufferer of this disease.

Despite having elevated calcium levels since 2010, I have been pushed from pillar to post. I'm either depressed, anxious, peri-menopausal, or a combination of all of these things. At no point did my endocrinologist suggest it could be anything else. In 2019 I suffered a fall and badly hurt my back, and subsequently developed neck and shoulder problems. Having tested my calcium levels again I was told I may have cancer. Then one nurse suggested maybe PHPT. This was dismissed until finally in October 2020 I was diagnosed with PHPT, after numerous scans, bloods and consultations.

Every area of my life has been affected by this disease. My relationship broke down and I'm now a single mother of triplets. My work has suffered to the point I may now be losing my job. My moods & awful temper has had a strain on my children and my lack of enthusiasm to do anything has in short, destroyed my life. I'm forty eight years old.

I was blessed and extremely fortunate to be accepted into the Hyperparathyroid UK Action4Change social media group and the wonderful Sallie Powell, without whom I would not have been referred to the amazing Shahab Khan and had my surgery in January 2021. The battle doesn't end here. Your body doesn't automatically repair years of damage in a heartbeat. Why is this situation so dire? Without this group of amazing people, many would be suffering in silence without their knowledge and support.

We are asking for an immediate update to the NICE guideline for PHPT published May 23rd 2019, to include those excluded based on calcium levels.

Also that there is a trained PHPT endocrinologist within each NHS Trust. This, I'm sure you will recognise will speed up the process regarding PHPT patients and also save the NHS so much funding!

Please listen to these stories. Please take on board these comments and please ensure there is change.

Regards

Claire Friend

Claire Holloway

Our Ref: SJP/SS-CEO NHS/15-03-21
Monday 15 March 2021

Dear Sir Simon Stevens,

RE: Action needed by NHS England for recognition & treatment of Hyperparathyroidism

I am writing to you as a member of Hyperparathyroid UK Action4Change, to tell you my story regarding Normocalcemic Primary Hyperparathyroidism.

It all started in 2001 when I was 13 years of age. I went to the doctors with a wide range of symptoms including change in bowel habits and severe lethargy. A blood revealed blood calcium level was slightly raised, which I only know now, because the endocrinologist who I have been under for three years told me when I was first referred to him.

From 2001 until 2018 my symptoms worsened. I had been to the doctors numerous times regarding my symptoms, calcium was slightly raised but nothing was ever done about the elevated levels. After years of trips to the doctors, with what was becoming debilitating symptoms, including heart palpitations, I decided to start researching my symptoms myself, and all roads led to hyperparathyroidism. With my newfound research I went back to the doctor who decided to do another calcium blood test. The blood results came back in line with my self-diagnoses and he referred me to the endocrinologist.

I have been under the Coventry University Hospital endocrine team for three years. For a year and a half of that, I was diagnosed with secondary hyperparathyroidism due to vitamin D deficiency. I corrected this deficiency with supplements and the endocrinologist team then went ahead with the relevant scans to find the adenoma. The adenoma was found on an ultrasound scan which actually wasn't for my parathyroids, it was for another issue with a lump in my neck.

All other scans were inconclusive. The endocrinologist referred me to the surgical team whilst monitoring my levels every three months.

In October 2020 I met with the surgeon. During this brief meeting we discussed the surgical procedure. This particular surgeon recommended medication and questioned if I needed the surgery, before refusing to do a four gland exploration due to risk to the vocal cords. I questioned having hyperplasia (multiple glands affected), his reply was 'the scans will direct me to which gland to operate on', even though they had been inconclusive. After speaking with the surgeon, the endocrinologist questioned if I needed the surgery as my last three calcium results were within range, even though the parathyroid hormone was still elevated.

Through the **Hyperparathyroid UK Action4Change** Facebook page, I came across a surgeon in Oxford who is broadening his knowledge on normocalcemic patients. He took me on as his patient under the NHS and removed a single three centimetre adenoma in January 2021.

Following my parathyroidectomy, my mental health has improved, and heart palpitations have ceased.

All of my symptoms could have been stopped before they started as well as NHS time and resources saved, if the GPs had been more informed about this disease, the endocrinologists had a wider knowledge of normocalcemic primary hyperparathyroidism and the surgical team didn't question all the information that had been supplied by a specialist.

If endocrinologists' followed the NICE guidelines, the cost to the NHS would be minimal, but due to lack of knowledge about this disease and the lack of commitment to operate on normocalcemic patients or actually many patients with primary hyperparathyroidism, the costs are mounting.

I appreciate your time to read my parathyroid story, and I hope you agree that change is needed to catch this disease in its early stages to end debilitating symptoms, and life-long damage to vital organs. I now have my life back, I am able to be the mum that I have always wished to be! Please help to give others the opportunity that I have been given.

Yours sincerely,

Claire Holloway

Colleen Jackson

Dear Sir Stevens

I am writing in support of letter reference SJP/55-CEONHS/15-0321 to share my experiences of Primary Hyperparathyroidism (PHPT), and my personal journey to get a diagnosis and treatment.

I am a member of Hyperparathyroid UK Action4Change, whose founder Sallie Powell, and other group members, have supported me throughout the last six years, with their knowledge and compassion.

I hope you will find the time to read this letter, and those of my fellow group members who have also written to you today, sharing their own experiences with the medical profession, whilst suffering with this debilitating disease.

Having been referred to the endocrinology department at Aintree University Hospital, Liverpool in 2015 after a bad fall, in which I fractured my pubic rami in three places, a DEXA scan revealed I had osteoporosis in my right hip and my back, and blood results showed raised calcium and parathyroid hormone (PTH) levels. I was diagnosed with Primary Hyperparathyroidism and began a three year "watch and wait" series of three monthly follow-up appointments, blood tests, negative ultrasound and nuclear scans, 3 annual bisphosphonate infusions for osteoporosis, and being constantly told by both Professor Cecil Thomas and his team that my raised calcium and PTH levels could not be causing the symptoms I described.

Eventually I arranged a private consultation with Mr Robert Hardy, endocrine surgeon. He examined me and looked at my blood results over the previous two years, listened to my history with this disease and the long list of symptoms I suffer with. He agreed to put me on his list for surgery if I could get endocrinology to refer me to him. I did this and having had a Cholestectomy in February 2018 for gall stones, I eventually had a parathyroidectomy on 27th September 2018, in which Mr Hardy removed a slightly enlarged Lipoadenoma.

Although my PTH dropped by fifty per cent during surgery, and the three remaining glands 'looked normal', follow-up blood tests revealed my calcium and PTH levels had not dropped and I was not cured. Professor Thomas refused to say if I could possibly have multi-gland disease, hyperplasia.

The 'watch and wait' continues, hampered by the current Pandemic, with four monthly telephone consultations with Professor Thomas. I am feeling really unwell again, my short term memory is now extremely poor and my balance is affected, as is my mood; it's as if 'the life has been sucked out of me' but coupled with nausea 24/7, gastric issues, bloated stomach, constant thirst, blurry eyes, headaches, sinus trouble, aching muscles and bones, weak grip (dropping things constantly) and repeated trips to the toilet, after trying to drink two to five litres of water to flush out the calcium every day. It is really difficult some days when you know a simple, short operation could cure you.

In September 2020, I had blood tests done at my GP surgery after a letter from endocrinology requested same. My calcium level was 2.8mmol/L, so my GP requested repeats, my calcium level had increased to 2.87mmol/L, a further test the following week revealed a calcium level of 2.89mmol/L, at which point my GP referred me to A&E on 13th October, after which I was admitted as an inpatient for saline and bisphosphonate infusion to lower my calcium and blood pressure. I was allowed to go home four days later, having also had a scheduled ultrasound for suspected pancreatitis.

As a result of the above, I was referred by Professor Thomas back to Mr Hardy whom I saw on 10th March 2021. He informed me that as my calcium was only just above normal at 2.68mmol/L (2.2-.60mmol/L) and the two nuclear scans I have just had, did not reveal an adenoma, he feels the chances of another failed parathyroidectomy are too high at the moment and he doesn't want to increase scar tissue/damage to my vocal chords, so I'm being referred back to endocrinology for regular bloods and to 'wait for the glands to grow'. I asked if the Pamidronate infusion could still be suppressing my PTH which he agreed, and although I expressed my concerns that this excess calcium is building up in soft tissues all over my body and major organs, and although maybe taking up to twenty years to kill me, I felt he had made his mind up. I left his office disappointed there would be no second operation and defeated as I've no fight left in me now, and I'm resigned to a slow painful *'bones, stones, groans and moans'* existence.

I have had many falls since suffering with this disease due to balance issues, fractured both my left and right ribs on separate occasions, broken toes, and fingers, and generally been regarded as clumsy having fallen down the stairs twice too. I have been diagnosed with a hiatus hernia, possible Barrett's Oesophagus (awaiting a date for follow up gastroscopy) taken Omeprazole for years to try and control the acid reflux, have a small 1cm abdominal hernia, osteoarthritis, prolapsed discs in my neck, depression or low mood, and itchy skin 'due to the menopause', and since that fall in November 2014, osteoporosis and peripheral neuropathy, and worsening cognitive function.

I was unaware I had a raised calcium level in 2006, which was never followed up. As this disease progressed, unknown to me, my fatigue, unclear thinking and not being able to physically climb several flights of stairs carrying patient files, or for trips to the toilet as my kidneys tried to flush out the excess calcium, took its toll and I reluctantly took early retirement in 2013 at aged sixty two years, from my wonderful NHS job, providing admin support to the Clinical team and Service Users of "The Rotunda Day Programme" run by Mersey Care NHS Trust. I feel this disease has robbed me of so much good health and happiness with my family, and friends, especially enjoying time with my soon to be retired husband of fifty years and our grandchildren. We had so many travel plans.

The amount of money for all this treatment and the medicines I have received over the last fifteen years, trying to get to a diagnosis and possible cure, is staggering, if one timely operation could have cured me of this cruel disease.

Why are so many PHPT patients still having to advocate for themselves, and to convince endocrinologists that their views are sometimes outdated? I would like a future where patients with this disease could receive better and speedier treatment from more informed endocrinologists, as a result of this condition being treated as a common endocrine disease, and given its own specialist doctors and surgeons. I am sure it would save the NHS so much money and reduce patient suffering.

Yours sincerely

Colleen Jackson

Dee Owen-Paxton

SJP/SS-CEO NHS/15-3-2

Re action needed by NHS England for recognition and treatment of hyperparathyroidism.

I am writing to you in support of the above reference as a member of Hyperparathyroid UK action group and a sufferer of this insidious disease.

I would like to tell you a little about my journey, hoping it will help you understand why we are approaching you, in the hope of updating the NICE guidelines.

I am a frontline worker in a pathology lab where we have been testing for Covid 19 as well as maintaining a routine service for two NHS hospitals and local GPs, and I have worked for the NHS for over thirty years.

I am a trained biomedical scientist specialising in medical microbiology, but I am now averaging four weeks off sick every six months and I struggle to do the job I know inside out. I can't remember names of bacteria and antibiotics, I can't answer phone queries because I forget where I am going with a sentence half way through it. I can no longer use a microscope all day as the pain in my joints and muscles prevents me. I lose my temper at nothing, I weep at nothing, and I am on report for my depressed attitude. My head hurts, my hands shake, I have to pee every hour, and I am exhausted. I can no longer participate in the on-call rota.

I have normocalcaemic primary hyperparathyroidism. However because my calcium falls below that quoted in the NICE guidelines my endocrinologist dismissed me back to my GP despite my PTH levels being three times higher than the top of the normal range.

I have attended A&E three times since being discharged from the endocrinologist, due to my symptoms, I've had many unnecessary tests and cost the NHS a lot of money. I approached a surgeon privately, the same one I had begged the endocrinologist and my GP to refer me to, and was immediately put on the surgical list because he is up to date and knowledgeable about PHPT disease.

Please consider our lobby, it will save a lot of people a lot of misery; a lot of employers a lot of sick pay; and most of all the NHS a lot of money.

Regards

D O-P

Dianne and Simon

Dear Sir Simon Stevens

I am writing to you, in conjunction with my wife, Dianne, who is a member of the Hyperparathyroid UK Action4Change support group. This letter is intended to give you a brief insight into our experience, of what transpired to be many years of misdiagnosis by the NHS, of the condition primary hyperparathyroidism.

To watch helplessly, as Dianne's health progressively deteriorated to such a level that she was no longer able to 'live' her life, but to simply 'exist', was nothing less than heart wrenching. Her muscles had become so weak that she was not able to walk at anything approaching a normal pace. It is no exaggeration to say that her step length was no greater than half the length of her own foot!

She found it incredibly difficult to perform basic everyday tasks, such as preparing a meal, as she did not have the physical strength and stamina to do such things as peeling and chopping vegetables or fruit, grating cheese, or stirring ingredients during the cooking process etc.

Because her muscles were so weak, she often found it impossible to do such simple things as opening some types of food packaging, particularly bottles, jars and cans, (both the "ring-pull" type, and those requiring the use of a can opener), having to rely on myself to do these tasks for her. She struggled to lift many items of cookware containing food, both during the cooking process and when serving, and was also unable to lift a full kettle of water in order to make hot drinks. General daily housework was something that she couldn't even contemplate, let alone carry out, and again, she relied heavily on myself to do these things for her.

Just having a shower each morning left her feeling totally drained of energy, and she even stated that her bath towel was beginning to feel too heavy for her to hold. Simply brushing her teeth became a difficult task, as her muscle weakness meant that she was unable to hold her arm in the same position, or exert pressure on her toothbrush, for any length of time. Literally everything she did became much more difficult, and took so much longer to do than normal.

When crossing a road, for example, she simply could not hurry, and just had to hope that drivers would be patient and considerate whilst she slowly tried to make it to the far kerb. Dianne's health eventually deteriorated to such an extent that we had to purchase both a wheelchair and a mobility scooter. Without these mobility aids she was unable to leave the house.

None of the GP's at our practice seemed to be listening to us, or taking our concerns about the ongoing deterioration in Dianne's health seriously. They didn't even appear to care very much that she was obviously suffering from a health condition that, for many years, was having a seriously negative impact on her quality of life, and indeed was continuing to do so. Instead, she was simply 'labelled' as having Chronic Fatigue Syndrome. Frankly, for several years, we both felt that we were 'banging our heads against the proverbial brick wall,' as we were getting absolutely nowhere, and Dianne's health was continuing to deteriorate. Quite honestly, we were both convinced that her health condition was the result of something other than Chronic Fatigue Syndrome, but none of our GP's were willing to investigate the situation further. We were constantly told that 'all the blood test results were normal.' It seemed that, as far as the GP's at our practice were concerned, Dianne had chronic fatigue syndrome, and that was that. No further action required!

Eventually, after much persistence on our part, we were able to persuade one of our GP's to finally agree to investigate Dianne's health condition further.

Despite being told, time after time, that 'all the blood test results were normal,' this transpired to be not strictly correct, as it was subsequently discovered, after further investigation, that the level of calcium in Dianne's blood was elevated.

Again, after further persistence on our part, Dianne was eventually referred to an endocrinologist, and it was during this consultation that we learned the level of calcium in her blood had been steadily rising, this having been the case over a period of the previous nine years!

Unbelievably, at the end of her consultation, Dianne was told by the endocrinologist, that there was 'no more he could do for her.' This statement led us both to further despair, as it appeared yet again, despite the blatant evidence, no further action was to be pursued and we had, once more, hit the proverbial 'brick wall.'

For several months Dianne received no further communication from any of the health professionals, and was just left in limbo. It subsequently transpired however, that the endocrinologist had, in fact, referred her to a parathyroid surgeon, and she had been placed on a waiting list for a parathyroidectomy. Dianne's operation was performed by an excellent parathyroid surgeon at one of our local hospitals here in Nottingham, in November 2020.

On the day, I watched as a nurse pushed her in a wheelchair along the corridor. The following day, after her operation, it was literally like a miracle had been performed overnight! She was now able to walk unassisted out of the hospital, at something resembling a more normal pace.

The transformation in her health, from one day to the next, was nothing less than remarkable! Thankfully, Dianne's health situation is now continuing to steadily improve, and she is starting to 'get her life back' again. As for me; Hallelujah; after many, many years, I now 'have my wife back,' instead of having to helplessly watch her slowly fading away to ultimately become little more than an empty shell.

It is almost beyond comprehension that, in this day and age, people are being forced to endure many years of a progressive deterioration in their health, along with the corresponding detrimental effect it has on their quality of life, (and the lives of their loved ones), before GP's and other health professionals eventually begin to listen to them, and start taking their concerns seriously.

In Dianne's case, as a direct result of continued misdiagnosis by the NHS, she has been slowly and progressively 'deprived' of over ten years of the ability to lead a normal life...

Ten years that she will never be able to retrieve.

Yours sincerely,

Simon

Dear Professor Amanda Howe

Campaign for the better recognition of Primary
Hyperparathyroidism (PHPT) - Our ref SJP/AH-RCGP/15-03-21

I am writing to you in support of Hyperparathyroid UK's campaign as above. I would like to share a part of my story to demonstrate this is a disease that is little understood or recognised by GPs. It is a degenerative disease for which the only cure is minor surgery. In reality I found GP's trivialised the progressive nature of this disease and there was little will on their behalf to put me their patient, forward for surgery, they seem content to watch and wait, to push pills and wait for end organ damage. In my case I have osteopenia and was heading for osteoporosis.

To briefly explain my story. For the last 15 years I have been presenting to my GP practice with various symptoms. I have had attempts to fob me off with depression, with menopause, with difficult to treat thyroid and that everything is age related. I have been sent for endless blood tests, investigations and to various consultants.

Having gained online access to my blood results I noted that I had (recent) below range phosphate, marked as abnormal. This had not previously been addressed. I took a call from a practice GP regarding my, relatively sudden, high blood pressure and cholesterol. During the last call I asked about the low phosphate level, the answer was "we don't worry about that". Now it doesn't take much knowledge or research to find that that these three issues are indicative of PHPT. If the GP had bothered to make that connection, if they had bothered to look at my calcium results which for years were either abnormally high or high normal, if they had bothered to link all my symptoms, then surely they could have made the connection themselves and ordered a test to confirm. Indeed they never actioned abnormally high Calcium going back to 2006.

As it was I flagged the low phosphate at an endocrinologist appointment soon after, they immediately made the connection asking to see Calcium results, suggesting it was long term undiagnosed PHPT and performing their own tests to confirm the diagnosis in Nov 2019.

With a diagnosis PHPT one would have thought the GP practice would act on that but no. The GP practise refused to refer me to a surgeon and said they couldn't (untrue).

I could go on at length regarding the battle I had but, suffice to say, I managed (despite non cooperative GPs and despite XXXXX CCG) to get a referral to a surgeon. In January this year I had a 3cm parathyroid tumour removed, with immediate relief of some of my symptoms and I am now cured of PHPT. Hopefully my osteopenia will now reverse.

That tumour has been there a long time wreaking who knows what damage.

I feel very sorry for patients who take their GP's word as gospel or who do not, for whatever reason, have the capacity to advocate for themselves and gain the appropriate treatment. I am sure there are many who have the disease but remain undiagnosed and are left with progressively worst damage to their bodies occurring. And many who are batting to get a diagnosis confirmed.

The NICE guidelines are ageist and also, arguably, sexist. In my experience, because I was over 50 years, I would have been left to get progressively more ill and unable to cope with day to day life - yet I work fulltime and was struggling.

What a revelation it has been to be cured, and what a difference it has made to my working life. The cost to the NHS and the country overall in terms of unnecessary medications, investigations and ill-health is shocking and needs to be taken into account. It is also appalling that no account is taken of the cost to individuals in dealing with disease, nor of the impact on quality of life of individuals. I work full-time but have struggled to do so whilst dealing with non-diagnosis, and then the battle for treatment, and as a consequence both my personal life and my career have suffered.

Question; why do GP's order blood tests but then not act on results marked abnormal?

Can you as President of the Royal Society of General Practitioners address the general lack of understanding of hyperparathyroidism, and also please take on board the issues I have raised, and use your influence to champion an update to the NICE Guidelines in the interest of patients. Thank you for reading, and please do not hesitate to contact me if you feel further detail of my personal experiences would be useful.

Yours sincerely

D Jones

15 March 2021
Our Ref: SJP/SS-CEO NHS/15-03-21

Dear Sir Simon Stevens

Campaign for the better recognition of Primary Hyperparathyroidism (PHPT)

I am writing in support of the above campaign and to give you a brief idea of the difficulties and problems I encountered in getting both diagnosis and treatment for PHPT.

I would like to briefly share a part of my story to demonstrate this is a disease that is seemingly little understood or recognised by GPs and Endocrinologists and also that the current NICE Guidelines are used to deny surgery when it is clearly needed.

PHPT is a degenerative, progressive disease but there is a cure - minor surgery. In my experience I found the disease is trivialised, despite the progressive nature of this disease. There was little will on the behalf of the medical practitioners to put me, their patient, forward for surgery. They seemed content to watch and wait, to push pills and wait for end organ damage. In my case I have osteopenia and was heading for osteoporosis.

To briefly explain my story. For the last 15 years I have been presenting to my GP practice with various symptoms. I have had attempts to fob me off with depression, with menopause, with difficult to treat thyroid and that everything is age related. I have been sent for endless blood tests, investigations and to various consultants.

Having gained online access to my blood results I noted that I had (recent) below range phosphate, marked as abnormal. This had not previously been addressed. I took a call from a practice GP regarding my, relatively sudden, high blood pressure and cholesterol. During the last call I asked about the low phosphate level, the answer was "we don't worry about that". Now it doesn't take much knowledge or research to find that that these three issues are indicative of PHPT. If the GP had bothered to make that connection, if they had bothered to look at my calcium results which for years were either abnormally high or high normal, if they had bothered to link all my symptoms, then surely they could have made the connection themselves and ordered a test to confirm. Indeed they never actioned abnormally high Calcium going back to 2006.

As it was I flagged the low phosphate at an endocrinologist appointment soon after. They immediately made the connection asking to see Calcium results, suggesting it was long term undiagnosed PHPT and performing their own tests to confirm the diagnosis in Nov 2019.

With a confirmed diagnosis of PHPT one would have thought the Endocrinologist and GP practice would act on that but no. The NICE guidelines were used to exclude me from surgery based on my age (56) and my calcium levels at the time, despite me being obviously biochemically diagnosed and obviously symptomatic (osteopenia). The GP practise refused to refer me to a surgeon and said they couldn't (untrue).

I could go on at length regarding the battle I had but, suffice to say, I managed (despite non cooperative GPs and despite XXXXX CCG) to get a referral to a surgeon.

 In January this year I had a 3cm parathyroid tumour removed, with immediate relief of some of my symptoms and I am now cured of PHPT. Hopefully my osteopenia will now reverse.

That tumour has been there a long time wreaking who knows what damage.

I feel very sorry for patients who take the word of consultants and GP's as gospel or who do not, for whatever reason, have the capacity to advocate for themselves and gain the appropriate treatment. I am sure there are many who have the disease but remain undiagnosed and are left with progressively worst damage to their bodies occurring. And many who are batting to get a diagnosis confirmed.

The NICE guidelines are ageist and it could be argued sexist. The failure of the guidelines to acknowledge normocalcemic PHPT is very damaging and I am a case in point. In my experience, because I was over 50 years, I would have been left to get progressively more ill and unable to cope with day to day life - yet I work fulltime and was struggling. What a revelation it has been to be cured and what a positive difference it has made to my working life. The cost to the NHS and the country overall in terms of unnecessary medications, investigations and ill-health is shocking and needs to be taken into account. It is also appalling that no account is taken of the cost to individuals in dealing with disease nor of the impact on quality of life of individuals. I work full-time but have struggled to do so whilst dealing with non-diagnosis and then the battle for treatment and as a consequence both my personal life and my career have suffered.

Question, why do GP's order blood tests but then not act on results marked abnormal?

Will you please consider and address the issues and suggestions in the letter sent by Hyperparathyroid UK ref SJP/SS-CEO NHS/15-03-2.

Thank you for reading and please do not hesitate to contact me if you feel further detail of my personal experiences would be useful.

Yours sincerely

D Jones

Elizabeth E Mitchell

Ref: SJP/SS-CEO NHS/15-03-21
15th March 2021

Dear Sir Simon Stevens

RE: Action needed by NHS England for recognition and treatment of Hyperparathyroidism

I believe GP's need educating about parathyroid as does A&E. My own GP didn't believe I had hyperparathyroidism despite my own research telling us it was so. He reluctantly sent off three referrals but as I found out much later, he put my lower results of calcium serum i.e. 2.59 and 2.62 on these, and that was why each was rejected as normal when I had readings of 2.68 and 2.62 that he should have shown.

I had to go private to prove I had the disease by which time my calcium level had gone up to 2.86. However even with this proof my GP then only sent me to an endocrinologist instead of straight to a surgeon. My level was 2.9 by time I had the operation 3 weeks ago. By then I had a renal stone and the start of osteoporosis. To add insult to injury my GP made the comments below on one of the referrals;

"I shall be most grateful for your help in managing this lady's beliefs and expectations regarding her quite fixed belief all her symptoms are related to her parathyroid, despite levels now being back in the normal range after starting Vit D3 1000iu daily. She is particularly fixated on her calcium levels, which historically runs at the upper end of the range."

The fact that A&E did not include calcium and PTH in their tests when I visit them twice in a week in the summer of 2018 having suffered two weeks of severe random stabbing pains all around my adnominal region every thirty seconds, night and day. They sent me home as suffering with constipation, which I had suffered for years (one of the symptoms of hyperparathyroidism).

The original symptoms changed to more pains in muscles and bones all around the body, though I still had regular adnominal pain, so more tests were done, a smear test, trans-virginal scan and MRI, Lyme disease test (I'm a volunteer in a garden where one of the other gardeners had the disease). Then as my ferritin level was still also high (430), and given my other symptoms, this resulted in tests at Kings College Hospital Haematology for porphyria and haemochromatosis (remarkably even they did not include PTH and calcium in their blood tests when they could not find an answer!) **I do not know how much was spent on these tests and consultations when all the while I suffered with primary hyperparathyroidism!**

It is not rocket science, once you have abnormal readings for PTH and calcium, you have an adenoma, in my case three, and only one showed up on the scan, they do not go away and only get worse causing damage in the meantime that could be avoided. Just cut them out and let people live their lives again. It breaks my heart when I read the cries for help on the support group site and I read the excuses their consultants give for not just getting on with the job that they know or should know will have to be done eventually.

I challenge you to find out how many people who had abnormal readings did not go on eventually to have a parathyroidectomy.

Elizabeth E Mitchell

Elizabeth Parry

Dear Amanda Howe

Re action needed by RCGP for recognition and treatment of primary hyperparathyroidism.

I am writing this letter to support Sallie Powell, CEO of Hyperparathyroid UK Action4Change.

I was finally diagnosed with normocalcemic primary hyperparathyroidism (NCPHPT), last September (2020) after eight years of investigations and tests. I had lived those years feeling very unwell, with constant nausea, unable to exercise to any extent, and a constant feeling of weakness.

I was sent for endoscopies and colonoscopies, and other tests over all these years, but nothing was ever diagnosed.

Two years ago I was diagnosed with severe osteoporosis in my spine (-3.5), at the age of sixty. Even then, the GP only ever tested calcium (not PTH), and because it was within range, ranted to start me on a bisphosphonate. I refused and spent a year trying to self-diagnose, eventually reading an article on normocalcemic primary hyperparathyroidism.

I asked my GP to test PTH, calcium and vitamin D in one blood draw, and sure enough, my parathyroid hormone levels were high.

I then saw Mr Shad Khan, Consultant Surgeon at Oxford University Hospitals who diagnosed NCPHPT. He operated in October 2020.

Five months on, my health has improved immeasurably, and I am slowly increasing my exercise regime. Sadly I am now left with severe osteoporosis, which could have been avoided if the NICE guidelines were correct, or if I had been diagnosed eight years ago.

All it would have taken was a simple blood draw of calcium, PTH and vitamin D, and recognition of the classification NCPHPT.

Please help us to get these guidelines changed.

Many thanks and kind regards

Liz Parry

Elisabeth White

Dear Sir Simon Stevens

Ref: SJP/SS-CEO NHS/15-03-21

RE: Action needed by NHS England for recognition and treatment of Hyperparathyroidism

You will have received a letter from Sallie Powell Founder/CEO of Hyperparathyroid UK, regarding the current guidelines and treatment of people with primary hyperparathyroidism.

This letter asks for your consideration regarding the following issues.

- The scale of misdiagnosis and misinformation to patients with primary hyperparathyroidism (PHPT), by many consultants, including endocrinologists, throughout the NHS, which causes prolonged treatment delays and can cause harm. We recognise the root is poor education at many levels throughout the NHS.

- We request an immediate update to the NICE guideline for PHPT, published 23 May 2019; https://www.nice.org.uk/guidance/NG132 to help many patients excluded by them based on calcium levels. We consider them to be a failure. They currently steer patients away from the NHS, towards private care, with their prohibitive surgical restrictions. Those without the option of private care are left to suffer dire consequences.

- Immense waste of NHS resources led by poor knowledge of PHPT. To quote Mr Shad Khan, Consultant Surgeon at Oxford University Hospitals; 'Studies looking at the cost effectiveness of parathyroidectomy compared to medical management show that surgery is far superior economically overall; **https://www.surgjournal.com/.../S0039-6060(16.../fulltext**

I would like to echo the effect that the following omissions in this guidance have had on the quality of life I experience as a wife who is tired all the time, as a mother of an eight year old who is in constant pain and sometimes crawls up the stairs at night on her hands and knees, at feeling so guilty when her eight year old has got out of bed to try to help her, as a fifty two year old woman who feels old before her time, who is loath to accept invitations as she will be too tired to actually converse or even be awake past 8 pm, and as a mental health nurse, who struggles with 'brain fog' and is trying to support patients and their carers who struggle with dementia (at least on this I can truly empathise);

- Information relating to two classifications of PHPT; normocalcemic PHPT and normohormonal PHPT. Both classifications require the same surgical cure as hypercalcemic PHPT.

- Post-operative care in the first days and months, which can lead to serious complications.

This illness is crippling and insidious as well as invisible and it is often an exhausting and arduous journey towards diagnosis and treatment. It feels that symptoms are dismissed, ignored and not understood.

My actual parathyroid journey began with a blood test in February 2019. After numerous visits to my GP with tiredness, poor sleep, aches and pains, depression and anxiety over several years, and after much research, I requested a rheumatology referral. I felt I had Fibromyalgia. At this appointment, routine blood tests discovered a high parathyroid hormone level; 18.48 pmol/l and raised calcium of 2.68 mmol/l leading to a referral to endocrinology.

In April 2019 the Endocrinologist noted I was a 'potential' candidate for a Parathyroidectomy, but that this may not be the cause of my symptoms as my calcium was only 'borderline raised'. Vitamin D was low so a review was made for four months, and I was prescribed supplements

September 2019, following investigations, a left parathyroid adenoma was discovered, and in October 2019 I was finally added to the surgical waiting list. Then obviously the pandemic hit, so eventually I had surgery in September 2020.

Throughout my journey I have felt as if I should not be as unwell as I have been because endocrinologists have consistently talked about my normal calcium level 'the relationship between hyperparathyroidism and symptoms is unclear especially when the level of hypercalcaemia is only mild' so when I saw the surgeon, he was a breath of fresh air and gave me confidence that I would feel better finally.

Following surgery in September 2020 I immediately felt better, my brain felt clearer and I felt like my zest for life had returned. This illness robs people of years of their lives, struggling with symptoms and/or diagnosis. My parathyroid hormone measured in surgery had reduced from 20.71 pmol/l to 6.57 pmol/l and considering I'd just had surgery I felt so much better.

In the months following my operation, I still remain tired at times, I still experience pain and aches in my bones, but this is nowhere near how I felt pre surgery. The brain fog is improved but not great, however the strategies I employ do help me function to some normality on some days. My PTH level continues to rise although nowhere near the level it was. My calcium remains the upper level of normal. The most dramatic change is in my mood, I am less anxious, most of my anxiety is around work and forgetting something, whereas before it was anything. I used to cry at 'the drop of a hat' and again this is improved. The suicidal thoughts are gone which I found was the most distressing aspect of this disease to me, as I have the most wonderful supportive family. Other diagnoses' are being considered currently but I do feel surgery has been beneficial.

Below, are excerpts from a letter I wrote in February 2020, illustrating how unwell I felt;

'I am struggling on a daily basis, the insomnia is awful and I am awake every night from 2-4 am. I am chronically tired, sometimes unable to climb the stairs. The feelings of anxiety are overwhelming and my short term memory remains very poor. I struggle to learn new things and my recall of recent events is very poor. I have palpitations and pain everywhere. My hair is falling out and my nails are very brittle. I am tearful irritable and short tempered which is very unlike me'

I am writing this letter of support for everyone who has this dreadful disease. I hope there can be more positive change in regard to care and management. It is a hidden disease and a disease I had not heard of prior to my diagnosis. More education is needed to prevent further suffering both mentally and physically.

I found this support group on Facebook and am consistently amazed at the level of knowledge and support of its members. Their knowledge around blood results, scans, supplements, surgery, care and treatment does, I feel put some of the medical profession to shame. Without them I would have 'drowned' and they have kept me 'afloat'

Kind regards and thanks in advance for your consideration

Elisabeth White

Encarnita Geddis

Our Ref: SJP/RS-Minister for Health-NI/15-03-21

Dear Robin Swann

Re: Action needed through the NHS in the UK for recognition and treatment of Hyperparathyroidism.

I, as a member of Hyperparathyroid UK Action 4 Change, am writing in support of the letter sent by Sallie Powell of Hyperparathyroid UK.

My story is too long, painful and hard to put into words but, because of the suffering of so many I would like to bring awareness of this misunderstood and little known disease.

On 23.07.2019, I was diagnosed with hypercalcemia in one of my multiple visits to A&E. Later on, a surgeon in Northern Ireland made the diagnosis of Primary Hyperparathyroidism.

In 1984 I had an anaphylactic reaction to an IVP Iodine based contrast. I was admitted to ICU but nevertheless, it was discovered the presence of calculi in both kidneys. I was diagnosed as well with chronic pyelonephritis. (Kidney stones are a sign of primary hyperparathyroidism), and from just there started my long path to hospital admissions with renal colic, pyelonephritis and lithotripsy sessions in Manchester and the City Hospital. Unfortunately, I ended up with kidney scarring and reduced kidney size in both kidneys. I am now at 3 CKD stage and my condition has deteriorated. I believe as many others do too, that my hypercalcemia has a lot to do with it.

Despite my kidney stone history no periodic calcium, PTH, Vitamin D tests seemed to have been done through the years. Calcium in blood fluctuates all the time and also needs to be checked along with parathyroid hormone PTH and vitamin D in the same blood draw to get a proper picture.

I will just list some of my other ailments:
1) High Cholesterol, 2) Hypertension, 3) diabetes, 4) 3 CKD stage, 5)

Thyroid nodules (Goitre), 6) I had a stomach stromal tumour removed, 7) a cholecystectomy, 8) multiple colon polyps, 9) tubular adenomas, 10) intramuscular lipoma in right tensor fasciae latae, which I still have, 11) Thalassemia minor was discovered by my doctor in the cholesterol clinic a few years ago.

I am vitamin D deficient and have low folic acid. It is hard for me to say how many of those complaints could be caused by high calcium in the blood. Although Hyperparathyroidism symptoms are far too numerous I will just mention a few:

a) bone pain, b) kidney stones, c) heart palpitations, d) chest pain, e) fatigue, f) insomnia, g) headaches, h) difficultly concentrating, i) memory loss, j) irritability, k) excessive hair loss, feeling rundown and low mood. I have suffered most of them.

Sometimes doctors have catalogued patients with this amount of symptoms as hypochondriacs but our suffering is very real. Hyperparathyroidism affects every cell of our bodies and if not discovered and treated early, the disease/condition will end up destroying every organ of our bodies. This is a progressive disease that could kill you at the end. A Parathyroidectomy is needed to cure all patients at all ages from this disease.

I believe I had this disease/condition for many years and have suffered enormously. The size of my adenoma could even have proved me right about the length of time I had the disease, according to my expert surgeon. I feel that I have been deprived of a proper and normal life which I have endured rather than have lived. I had forced myself to keep working and keep going in spite of how unwell I felt.

For many years before my parathyroidectomy I ended up many times in A&E and at my GPS surgery with heart palpitations, chest pains, raised BP and generally feeling very unwell. I collapsed in a veterinary Hospital and was rushed and admitted to hospital but unfortunately, nothing was discovered.

Sallie Powell, and all of us in our group, want to raise awareness of this devastating disease which cripples lives and makes other people so ill they cannot cope with their lives. I had a parathyroidectomy and I was told that I was cured. Many of my previous symptoms have gone and surgery stops the progression of the disease.

Unfortunately, the damage already caused by the disease for so many years has left me with health issues which are irreversible.

It is because of the suffering of people diagnosed, and undiagnosed with this disease, that more knowledge of this condition is desperately needed. Finding this disease early is paramount to halt suffering for us all.

Yours faithfully

Encarnita Geddis.

Eve Thirkle

Dear Sir Simon

RE: Action needed by NHS England for recognition and treatment of Hyperparathyroidism

I am writing today to support the Founder/CEO of Hyperparathyroid UK, established in September 2014. I am asking you to read this letter and others being sent to you today regarding the following three issues, namely:

1. The scale of misdiagnosis and misinformation to patients with primary hyperparathyroidism (PHPT), by many consultants, including endocrinologists, throughout the NHS, which causes prolonged treatment delays and can cause harm. There seems to be poor education at many levels throughout the NHS. There needs to be a trained PHPT endocrinologist within each NHS Trust. This would speed up the process regarding PHPT patients and also save the NHS so much funding!

Fully trained staff with a greater understanding is the key here

2. The failure of the NICE guidelines for PHPT, published 23 May 2019, to help many patients. A large number of patients are excluded from treatment based solely on calcium levels.

The guidelines should place more emphasis on the reciprocal interaction between calcium and PTH and also the possibility that patients may have either normocalcaemic or normohormonal primary hyperparathyroidism presentations.

The present guidelines fail many patients with their prohibitive surgical restrictions of requiring very high levels of calcium before referral to surgery. They currently force many patients away from the NHS and having to seek private care. Those unable to utilise the option of private care are left to suffer life limiting consequences.

3. Immense waste of NHS resources (and wider) is occurring, occasioned by poor knowledge of PHPT. Patients with calcium levels judged to be below those who need a surgical referral from the NICE guidelines are struggling to hold down their jobs, manage themselves and their families and often can no longer be productive members of society but have to rely on disability benefits.

To quote Mr Shad Khan, Consultant Surgeon at Oxford University Hospitals; 'Studies looking at the cost effectiveness of parathyroidectomy compared to medical management show that surgery is far superior economically overall'

I am writing to you as a member of the action group Hyperparathyroid UK and as a sufferer of this disease. My own journey is chronicled below. My treatment (or rather lack of it) is under investigation by the Ombudsman at present.

Thank you for your time in this matter

E. Thirkle

My Primary Hyperparathyroid Journey

I experienced worsening and wide-ranging symptoms over a period of nearly two years. These symptoms escalated in the spring and summer of 2018, resulting in blood tests and a consequent referral to Endocrinology. My GP said these results were indicative of Primary Hyperparathyroidism and referred me to see an endocrinologist. He referred me to the https://patient.info/ site and their information leaflets as well as the uptodate.com website.

The chronology and history of blood tests and ongoing symptoms were detailed by me in a patient history document along with a chart of blood test results. These documents were given as copies to the endocrinology registrar when I saw him in July 2018 for my endocrinology assessment. When I received a copy of my notes under a Patient Access request I was surprised to see that these did not form part of my clinical record.

My full biochemistry results clearly documented both elevated calcium with inappropriately suppressed PTH, along with calcium at the high end of normal concurrent with a PTH at the high end of normal too. The normal homeostatic mechanism clearly was not working correctly.

Information provided by my GP made it clear that if calcium is high, PTH should be low and vice versa. *'High concentrations of serum calcium inhibit PTH secretion, while low concentrations stimulate it'* is from supporting document "Patient Info Leaflet on Hyperparathyroidism" This makes it clear that high (or top of the range) calcium in a non-suppressive relationship with high (or top of the range) PTH is not normal. As a retired radiographer this was confirmed by advanced physiology textbooks in my possession.

This had been recognised by my GP, however the endocrinology registrar failed to recognise this non-suppressive relationship until I highlighted it to the clinician myself, whereupon he acknowledged that this could possibly be due to a parathyroid issue.

During the consultation my husband and I were shocked and surprised regarding how little he appeared to know about hyperparathyroidism. Indeed, it was embarrassing to have to explain the condition to him. We had questions which he struggled to answer. I was sent for further blood tests.

These blood test results clearly documented (yet again) elevated calcium with inappropriately suppressed PTH.

I then received a copy of a letter from the registrar in which he stated both that the hypercalcaemia was resolved but also that this conclusion was not borne out by the calcium levels on 27th July 2018. One of these conclusions must have been incorrect. I was sent for further urine and blood tests.

In the interim I had several visits to A&E with several musculoskeletal issues relating to the hypercalcaemia.

I heard nothing further from the endocrinology team after the blood and urine tests performed at the end of August, but received a letter out of the blue on 10th September cancelling my follow-up appointment of 21st January 2019. When I rang to see if another appointment was being arranged I was told that I had been discharged, but the admin person I was speaking to, had no further details.

After this I then received a letter from the registrar stating that the most recent test had shown a normal calcium result (2.52 upper quartile) along with a normal PTH (6.2 upper quartile) and a normal urinary calcium excretion of 7.3 mmol/24h (again upper quartile). He stated in this letter that due to all these normal results he was discharging me from the endocrine clinic. In doing so, the registrar continued to show a lack of understanding of the negative feedback loop of PTH and calcium.

If you take each result in isolation it would imply that there was no issue and that everything was 'normal'. However, when an upper quartile level of PTH sits beside an upper quartile calcium result it indicates a non-suppressive relationship between calcium and PTH. The lack of understanding of this relationship by the registrar and his seniors has led to a failed diagnosis and possible harmful progression of the effects of hyperparathyroidism.

These levels should have led the registrar and his superiors to further investigations rather than dismissing all results as 'within the normal range' and discharging me from the service. There was no advice for the GP to monitor my calcium in future.

By the end of October my muscle and ankle pain combined, had led to my needing to walk with a stick. I was struggling so much with climbing stairs that my husband and I were considering adding a second bannister to assist me in using the stairs.

My continuing symptoms meant that I had to reduce my workload. When completing my availability on my calendar for work I had to request a maximum of 2 days of work to be allocated each week rather than being available for 3 or 4 days. As I only get paid for the days that I work this had an effect on my income. This placed a significant cost on myself and my family.

When I approached my GP regarding the worsening of my symptoms and the possibility of a second opinion I was told that because of the letters from the endocrinology team, I did not need any more referrals or blood tests.

I consequently began some research of my own into how to obtain a second opinion. I discovered that there is no legal right to a second opinion and my GP was within his contractual duties to refuse a further referral.

I had been left in limbo with the symptoms that I had of feeling 80 years old but not yet 60. This is the point at which I began researching the possibility of a private consultation. I also queried the discharge with the hospital via PALs which led to an unsatisfactory phone call with the consultant endocrinologist – never recorded in my hospital notes – which also seemed not to register the issue of the reciprocal relationship between PTH and Calcium.

Acting on recommendations via the Hyperparathyroid UK support group, I was successful in seeing a clinician privately who diagnosed primary hyperparathyroidism from exactly the same blood test results seen by the endocrinology team in my local hospital. Following private scans and private surgery, two hyperplastic glands were removed, and my aches and pains, stiffness and many other symptoms were relieved within days of the operation. This cost me over £8000 from my savings.

Gill

Dear Sir

Our Ref: SJP/AG-CEO NHS/15-03-21 - RAISING AWARENESS OF PRIMARY HYPERPARATHYROIDISM

I felt moved to write in support of the above letter, with my own experience of primary hyperparathyroidism.

Back in 1992 my son suffered, at 6 days old, neo-natal tetany, He was admitted as an emergency, underwent all sorts of invasive tests but was eventually diagnosed, put on a drip and was discharged after forty eight hours. We learnt that this had been caused by very low calcium levels.

Consequently, my own calcium levels were tested, and found to be at the top of the range, but 'normal'. Sixteen years later, as I was waiting for a cholesterol test at my local surgery, I saw the words 'probable primary hyperparathyroidism' on my notes from 1992 and queried it with the nurse, since I hadn't heard of it.

She had to look it up. We decided to check my calcium again and a further blood test was ordered, which showed that it was indeed very high by this time.

I was referred to endocrinology, and then to surgery quickly, which was funded through a health insurance policy at work. I had three adenomas removed in two operations.

Due to the lack of follow-up at the initial stages of this condition, despite someone actually recognising what the problem was, I now have kidney stones, osteoporosis, nephrocalcinosis and many other symptoms of primary hyperparathyroidism.

I really believe we need to re-educate regarding this condition, both at primary care level and in endocrinologists and their registrars.

The NICE guidelines are also prohibitive in terms of surgery for patients with what is referred to as 'mild' primary hyperparathyroidism, when all the research and evidence shows that symptoms and end-organ damage do not correlate with calcium levels.

Thank you for the time taken to read this – I hope it will serve to highlight our need for intervention which I believe will help thousands of struggling patients and, indeed, save some money for our wonderful NHS.

Yours faithfully

Gill

Guy Smith

Ref: SJP/SS-CEONHS/15/03/21

Dear Sir Simon,

I am writing in support of the letter sent to you by Sallie Powell, referenced above, and wish to describe my own experience of attempting to be either diagnosed with Primary hyperparathyroidism (PHPT), or to have it ruled out. There lies the problem.

I have been ill for 15 years. Eventually diagnosed with M.E./Chronic Fatigue Syndrome. The cumulative effect of this illness on my life has been devastating. I lost a career I worked very hard to establish, together with my independence, pension and a self-determined future. ME/CFS is a 'diagnosis of exclusion'. Many medics believe it has a psychological basis. I have generally been encouraged to learn to live with symptoms and limitations. I have always doubted the diagnosis but in my experience, it is a pigeon hole that is difficult to escape from. Few people will listen, let alone believe you.

A few years ago I discovered quite by chance that I had high calcium blood test results. Something I was never told about by my GP practice. Personal research quickly flagged up primary hyperparathyroidism as a possible cause.

The GPs I saw knew next to nothing about the condition so I requested a referral to an endocrinologist. Having been warned that the NHS waiting list was anything up to a year (pre-pandemic), I decided to pay for a private consultation. I looked for an endocrinologist and found one who stated parathyroid disease as an interest. After a number of tests I was told I didn't have the disease. The reasons given didn't tally with what I had learnt through fairly basic research. Surely though a consultant level doctor working for both the NHS and in private practice would know? Apparently not.

I was left unsure of what to do next or who to turn to, for help and advice. There are excellent specialist clinics with informative websites in the United States but it is somewhat difficult to access diagnosis and treatment when you live in Brighton, UK. They however, see the problem frequently faced by many patients in the UK. I managed to find the website and Facebook group Hyperparathyroid UK Action4Change, and voiced my concern about my negative diagnosis. Other members quickly came forward to confirm similar experiences with the same endocrinologist. They had gone on to be correctly diagnosed elsewhere and surgically cured - in some cases at considerable personal cost.

What quickly became clear, was that this is not an isolated case of encountering a consultant who is poorly educated, but is in fact, worryingly widespread. This letter, therefore, is not a complaint about an individual. It is an earnest plea to investigate what is going wrong with the training and accreditation of UK endocrinologists. I don't believe it is an issue of differing medical opinion or a doctor's personal approach.

On a daily basis, people are finding their way to the group and coming forward with stories where what they have been told, is demonstrably wrong. It seems there is a lack of standards set via continued professional development and accreditation, as well as inadequate NICE guidelines which exclude countless people, who in fact have the same disease. My understanding is, intervention from the top can begin to change this situation.

I may or may not have parathyroid disease. I still don't know. I do however need to have faith and confidence that any diagnosis made is correct. At this point in time, I simply do not.

Hyperparathyroidism is not vanishingly rare, it is the third most common endocrine disease. It is not, for many people, the 'mild' disease many medics describe it as. The neglected suffering of individuals aside, the cost to the NHS of treating symptoms and worsening disability caused, must be immense.

I believe the NHS is currently failing a significant group of patients. It should not be up to (very ill) individuals to scrabble around looking for professional help, they can actually trust. I hate to think how many people have failed to get an accurate diagnosis or have accepted that no action (surgical intervention) is required. My understanding is, they will continue to have blighted lives and early deaths. Primary Hyperparathyroidism is CURABLE when correctly diagnosed and treated. The ONLY treatment is surgery.

Thank you for taking the time to read this. I hope you can offer some support and look into the issue.

Regards

Guy

Heather Burns

Dear Amanda

I am writing to you as a member of the excellent Hyperparathryoid UK Action4Change group. Our CEO Sallie Powell has sent you a letter reference SJP/AH-RCGP/15-03-21 regarding the action needed by NHS England and RCGP for recognising and treating hyperparathyroidism. A copy of this letter has also been sent to Sir Simon Stevens.

Here is my story re diagnosis problems and appropriate treatment.

In 2006 following a routine blood test before a colonoscopy, I was found to have a high calcium and subsequently it was found my parathyroid levels were raised too. I was diagnosed with primary hyperparathyroidism. I was seen by a local endocrinologist and referred to a general surgeon with an interest in parathyroid surgery. No scans or pre-operative assessments were made prior to surgery and potential removal of any enlarged large parathyroid glands. I was led to believe I had one parathyroid removed.

Ten years later when I requested my surgery notes I found none had been removed. I later found he only did ten parathyroid surgeries a year which to me does not demonstrate a great deal of experience in parathyroid surgery. The surgeon then dismissed me from his care when I did not feel any better and referred me to someone who I was led to believe was an endocrine doctor – he turned out to be a general medical doctor with an interest in endocrine disorders. I say this because I feel all patients with hyperparathyroidism deserve to be seen by specialist endocrinologists who are proactive in their care and treatment.

I was seen three monthly initially and had recurrent blood tests, at significant cost to the NHS. My parathyroid and calcium levels remained high and I was experiencing symptoms of acute tiredness, brain fog, bone pain (something I would not like anyone to experience), and gastric problems. I continued to work as a nurse four days a week, but this drained my energy so my social life vanished. Even when just ironing I would need to rest every so often. I used to say to my husband "That's it, I cannot do anymore, I need to sit down." When my children came around I often felt so tired that I was going to pass out. Not a life just an existence. It was recommended I start taking Cinacalcet.

Cinacalcet was then a new drug of choice, meant to be used short term to regulate calcium levels and was very costly for the NHS. I could only get it from Manchester Royal Infirmary initially, until at a later stage my GP was asked to fund it. This medication had some effect on relieving my symptoms, but I was unaware of the damage the long term effect of having hyperparathyroidism was having on my body. In 2012 I was diagnosed as having osteopenia _ the next step if this disease continued to drain calcium from my body - was osteoporosis. However I was not offered any change in treatment nor was it suggested I have a re-op. I regularly travelled to Manchester, an hour away from my home, for outpatient appointments in a clinic very oversubscribed. This meant I was there for several hours at a time, and as time for consultations was very limited, nothing changed. At one stage my Cinacalcet medication was raised so I was on the top dose I could take but still no suggestion of a referring me back to a surgeon. This continued for ten years until I decided to educate myself on my condition and see if I could change things.

So I joined Sallie's Facebook site Hyperparathyroid UK Action4change. What an eye opener - I became aware of the danger the high parathyroid hormone and calcium levels were doing to my body, and I was supported and empowered to take things into my own hands. Through the site I was able to gain information on reputable surgeons who were specialised in re-ops. I arranged to see Mr Palazzo in London for a private appointment. He agreed to consider me for surgery subject to scans etc. He also contacted my GP to make a referral to him as an NHS patient. I subsequently had various investigations and scans all in London. Mr Palazzo wasn't sure he could help me by surgery but was prepared to try. As he carries out 142 surgeries a year and specialises in re-ops I put my confidence in him – my last hope really of a cure from this dreadful disease. Thankfully my surgery was successful and the rogue parathyroid was discovered during difficult surgery during which half my thyroid was removed. My recovery however, has been very slow – they say at least a month for every year you have the disease – and I still have osteopenia, Interestingly since surgery my angina (due to cardiac syndrome X) has significantly improved. As have my headaches and palpitations, so I assume that the calcium had an impact on all of those symptoms too.

I am sure you will agree I have cost the NHS a significant amount of money over the years. My big concern is that every day I read stories from people who cannot get the surgery they desperately need. Many doctors are ill informed on hyperparathyroidism and do not realise how it limits our lives and causes long term damage to our bodies. I would like to see everyone empowered to change things for themselves but we have to realise this is not possible. Therefore, they all need access to the best possible care wherever they are and access to competent and knowledgeable endocrinologists and parathyroid surgeons.

Thank you for taking the time to read my letter. I enclose a copy of Sallie's letter which will give you more information on our hope to improve the diagnosis and treatment of Hyperparathyroidism.

Kind regards

Heather Burns.

Helen

Dear Sir Simon Stevens,

Re: Action needed by NHS England for recognition and treatment of Hyperparathyroidism - Ref: SJP/SS-CEO NHS/15-03-21

I am writing as a member and user of the support group Hyperparathyroid UK – Action4Change, to add weight to the request for action, to raise awareness for the recognition and treatment needs of patients with Hyperparathyroidism.

I was diagnosed last year when a follow up cholesterol check showed raised levels of calcium in my blood. The test was repeated with the same result. The locum GP told me not to ask her anything about what this might mean for me, as she didn't know, but she was referring me to an endocrinologist who could answer my questions.

A few months later I had a telephone consultation with the endocrinologist who told me he was referring me for two scans (nuclear and Ultrasound) and would ask my GP to arrange a DEXA scan once the machine was working again. He asked if I felt well. I said pretty much. I believe this led to him writing to my GP that I had very asymptomatic Primary Hyperparathyroidism. However, had I known about the disease, I would have informed him that I have high blood pressure, raised cholesterol, joint pain, insomnia (averaging 5 hours sleep a night for many years), some memory loss and concentration problems, hot flushes and heart racing, feeling completely overwhelmed by small challenges, impacting on the final years in my career and resulting in my early retirement.

I had put all these things down to stress and post-menopausal symptoms that some unlucky women just have to put up with. From my own research I now know that some of these symptoms could well be due to consequences of having Hyperparathyroidism. The bone density scan has shown I also have osteoporosis. I am 65, so it seems likely this has also been caused or certainly contributed to by Hyperparathyroidism.

The endocrinologist told my GP (a different one, as the locum had left) to prescribe me Alendronic Acid. At that stage he wanted to monitor my calcium levels every six months. The conversation I thought we would have after the tests did not seem to be on offer anymore, so I wrote to him. I told him I was distressed to learn over the phone from my GP that I had osteoporosis and that I had reservations about taking Alendronic Acid. Further, I asked why the symptoms/result of the illness were being treated when the cause could be removed, at which point the symptoms would hopefully improve. The endocrinologist rang me and said that since having more test results he would be referring me to surgery.

The test results have shown:
Raised calcium levels
Raised parathyroid hormone levels
Raised potassium levels
Low vitamin D level (for which he recommended a supplement).
Osteoporosis in femoral neck and osteopenia at other test points

I was prescribed Alendronic Acid, which I was anxious about. Clearer advice about use in cases of Hyperparathyroidism would be helpful. There is research showing that over time the bones may be denser, but hip fracture numbers are actually increased when compared to no medication. I was also concerned that they might alter the bone structure so that it was more difficult to repair when my bones reverted to absorbing calcium after surgery.

Having said I would be referred for surgery, instead the team decided I should have a CT scan. I was lucky to get a cancelation slot very quickly. After a few weeks I emailed the consultant to ask if this had given more detail so I could now proceed to surgery and that if it hadn't, requesting I be referred for surgery by a surgeon experienced in four gland exploration.

It has been very helpful having access to the information available through Hyperparathyroid UK – Action 4 Change. Without the group I would have been ignorant about the NICE Guidance for Hyperparathyroidism and what I could hope to expect, by way of treatment and referral. This knowledge has enabled me to make more informed decisions as well as what questions to ask and what reasonable expectations might be. I believe that this has helped move things along and I have just been told that I have been referred for surgery.

The Guidance does not give much specific information about aftercare e.g. calcium supplements and I understand from reading other people's experiences that this is an important consideration. In addition although my readings have given clear indication for a diagnosis, others without classic systematic reference points have struggled to get the disease recognised and/or taken seriously.

I was surprised that I had never heard of this debilitating and damaging disease as I have considered myself interested and alert to issues relating to women's health. The profile needs to be raised at primary health care level. I am enormously grateful to the locum GP who, as part of a routine test checked my calcium level and referred me to an Endocrinologist. However I have no idea how long I might have had this condition, and she was the first to admit she knew nothing about what having raised calcium might mean – "so don't ask me any questions".

When I read other people's experiences I suspect I am one of the luckier ones. Even so I have been significantly affected by this disease and the sooner it is more widely known about, recognised and diagnosed with a clear and unambiguous route to treatment and recovery the better. Indeed, letting people struggle for years with the various ailments they suffer and need to seek remedy for, puts a long term heavy toll, not only on the overall welfare of those people and their families, but on the health service.

Yours sincerely

Helen

Jackie Baldwin

Our Ref: SJP/SS-CEO NHS/15-03-21

Dear Mr Stevens

I am writing in support of the Hyperparathyroid UK Action4Change support group which has literally been my lifeline with this awful condition.

For many months leading up to October 2018, I had suffered with differing symptoms from memory issues, heartburn, anxiety, severe fatigue, brain fog and excruciating joint pain in both my arms and legs. After being told by my usual GP that it was probably 'my age', I finally found a GP who took my concerns seriously and ordered some blood tests. Her opinion was that I probably had PHPT and would need surgery to cure it. This was a relief on one hand and a scary thought on the other, at the thought of possibly having to undergo surgery. I was however, reassured to get an appointment to see a specialist in April 2019.

However, nothing prepared me for the next few months and the battle I had to fight to get an endocrinologist (*the expert!*) to accept that I did indeed have PHPT.

My initial consultation was a list of about twenty questions regarding symptoms. I answered yes to every question except one and because of this I was told that as I hadn't answered yes to **all** of the symptoms, in their opinion, I didn't have the condition and he ordered more blood tests and prescribed a high dose of vitamin D to 'manage' the situation.

I now know that with this condition you can have just some or all of the symptoms and I also know that this condition simply cannot be managed; **the only cure is surgery to remove the adenoma that is causing the issues.** I left in tears feeling totally deflated and then waited another three months for the next appointment.

At the next appointment (same endo) my vitamin D levels were still low and my calcium levels were still high, yet still I was told that these levels were 'relatively normal' I didn't have PHPT, and that I would be referred to rheumatology for further investigations.

I went back to my GP who was very supportive and insisted I have another appointment with an endocrinologist. Another three months later and I met a different endocrinologist who was the complete opposite. His opening line to me was *"we need to arrange for you to have scans and then surgery as this is the only option here"*. I looked at him with absolute incredulity and said *"are you saying that I have PHPT?"* and he said *"oh yes, without a shadow of a doubt, 100 percent"*.

Although very relieved that I had finally got a proper diagnosis, I was very angry that I had been 'fobbed off' by the previous endo. How can two specialists working in the same field have such differing opinions and lack of basic knowledge??! If the first endo had not been so ignorant of basic facts then I would not have had to endure months of agony and been left in a dire financial situation due to not being able to do my job.

After joining the PHPT Support Group, I learned that that this is happening all over the country and patients are being made to feel that their illness is in their minds. It is truly shocking.

I finally got my surgery in March of 2020 and was told by the surgeon that I would be back to normal within weeks. Wrong again! It can take many months for your body to recover and for your bones to re-mineralise, and then only with supplements, none of which were even mentioned to me by either the endo or the surgeon.

I only found this information out after joining the support group and getting advice off people who had been through the same circumstances and who have a far superior knowledge of this disease than most of the so-called professionals. It makes me extremely saddened (and angry) to think how many other people are going undiagnosed or misdiagnosed and are living with no quality of life when they could get treatment and recover if it were not for the ignorance of so many medical professionals.

To finish, I would like to say that just over a year after surgery, I am not yet fully recovered and still suffer with some pain and fatigue. If it were not for the knowledge of the Hyperparathyroid UK Action4Change Support Group and their advice re supplements and diet, I truly feel I would be in a very dark place now, if here at all.

This disease has truly debilitated me in a way I never thought possible and I feel strongly that the whole medical profession (and especially endocrinologists) need to be made more aware of the effects of this condition and therefore not be condemning people to a life of pain and misery through sheer ignorance.

I fully support Sallie Powell and her amazing work for all PHPT sufferers and I truly hope that people sit up and take note.

Yours Sincerely

Mrs J Baldwin

Jackie Ribeiro

Dear Sir Simon,

Thank you for all you have done in your acting role as CEO for the NHS in these unprecedented times. It is much appreciated by everyone. As a former teaching midwifery sister I wish that I had been well enough to help my community more, especially to volunteer in the vaccine role out.

My life has been blighted by hyperparathyroidism, at first insidiously, in my early forties. I am now sixty two years old. As it is the third most common endocrine disorder in the UK I have been astounded at how it is mismanaged by endocrinologists when a quick route to a cure is a fairly simple operation (parathyroidectomy) to remove the offending tumours which draw calcium out of our bones with dire systemic consequences for our bodies.

My early symptoms were put down to the peri-menopause in my early forties even though I was skeptical as I am a toughie used to running a labour ward efficiently, and had gone on to change career teaching A levels to lively and challenging teenagers.

My symptoms stepped up six months after I tragically lost my husband. He was a GP and I found him after he had committed suicide. I had to keep it together for my young children's sake, and I went back to work promptly as I had students about to sit their A level exams. I was told that my stomach, muscle, sleep disturbance, tinnitus, and bone pains were an effect of PTSD. I refused to take antidepressants as I was coping psychologically.

Fast forward sixteen years, as I don't want to bore you with the endless consultations, bloods tests and scans; I am waiting for my third parathyroidectomy. This time I have a lovely surgeon, Mr. Khan, at Oxford University Hospitals, who acknowledges calcium levels fluctuate with this disease, so that you get the odd day of feeling 'alright'. For the last few years my symptoms have been dire, and a member of our support group who caught Covid has likened her symptoms to that of post Covid. Personally I liken it to having gastric flu three or more times a week, accompanied with bone pain. You feel as if you are literally being poisoned.

I feel angry for the countless times I have been put down by so called health professionals who have delayed my cure. I had my first op privately, in January 2017 out of desperation, and a tumour that was twenty five times the size of a normal gland was removed. That operation cost me half of my small NHS pension lump sum. It made me feel sad that my children hadn't had the best of me during their informative years, as well as not having their father to guide them.

My second parathyroidectomy scheduled at Gloucester, over two years later (after Calcium levels rose again) was cancelled twenty minutes before it was due to take place, as my pre-op calcium level had dropped. The surgeon thrust a letter under my nose in front of his team, composed by an endocrinologist who I had never met, to say that she didn't think I had a return of the disease. I had been nil by mouth since five am, and was all gowned up for theatre. Eight months later, I had a second adenoma removed, which was stuck to my oesophagus at Oxford university Hospitals, after being referred there by a lovely lady surgeon in Warwick whose scan showed the likely adenoma was in my chest. I took slight gratification in writing to the surgeon in Gloucester to inform him, as he had told me I that I had 'Globus Hystericus' when I complained of feeling a lump when I swallowed.

Just as we went into lockdown, I was informed that I would need a third op as my calcium levels had risen yet again, and I am still waiting. I have also passed kidney stones, at home alone. An awful experience to go through. Unfortunately I am a rare case where three glands have developed tumours and two are ectopic, in the wrong place.

I feel sad and sickened for all the members of our group who have the experience of dealing with some of these so called health professionals, especially the endocrinologists. Also that it has been such a waste of my career. I hope that I can do some sort of volunteering work after this nightmare is over.

There has to be a clearer way to diagnose this disease. This would save the government so much money in the long run. Especially as grimly, a lot of people go undiagnosed with this disease and die of its undetected consequences, namely dementia, osteoporosis and cardiac issues.

I myself now have osteoporosis, memory issues and cardiac complications. I am hoping that I can arrest their progression after this third and final operation. In total over the last few years my care has involved eleven scans, eight of which have been nuclear, endless GP consults, physio appointments and treatment for a fractured foot. Some GPs have quite shamefully gas lighted me. Also I have seen cardiologists, and a neurologist because they put some symptoms down to MS. The neurologist suggested that I go away and get on with my life. My dear husband would have been horrified.

This is not how I planned to spend my retirement and I am angry because it needn't have been like this.

I really hope that as your tenure as CEO of the NHS comes to an end you will not put this pile of letters in the drawer of your desk and walk away. Our objective is that the NICE guidelines are revised to hasten diagnosis of this cursed disease.

Also a simple screening of calcium levels for adults would help detect and monitor people more effectively. In fact, they did do that in Gloucestershire about five years ago for over fifty fives', but the surgeon said he put a stop to it as too many were being picked up!

It is best to detect this disease early, rather than wait for end organ damage at huge cost to the NHS. Also, most importantly, good health cannot be quantified in monetary terms. That is one thing that this awful pandemic has demonstrated. There are names and lives that make up the statistics.

Take care and thank you for reading my letter. I wish you the very best regarding all you do in the future.

Yours sincerely

Jackie Ribeiro (Mrs.)

Jane Church

A letter has also been sent to Professor Amanda Howe by email

Dear Sir Simon Stevens

Re: Recognition of Primary Hyperparathyroidism

I am writing in support of letter reference **SJP/SS-CEONHS/15-0321** to share my experience of Primary Hyperparathyroidism. I understand a number of my colleagues will be writing to you and I hope you can take the time to read my story.

I was diagnosed with Primary Hyperparathyroidism in October 2019 after suffering with the condition for an unknown period of time, but it is likely that I had been experiencing symptoms for the previous three years. Prior to suffering with PHPT, I had been in good health. As you know, the condition Primary Hyperparathyroidism is caused by one or multiple parathyroid gland(s) malfunctioning causing too much calcium in the blood and urine. The condition has multiple symptoms, including:

- Bone pain
- Muscle pain
- Bone and muscle weakness
- Brain fog
- Anxiety
- Depression
- Kidney stones and more general kidney issues

The longer someone goes undiagnosed with the condition, the more damage is being done to their body internally (bone fragility, kidney damage etc.) and the longer it will take the individual to recover if they are fortunate enough to get into the system and, ultimately, be referred to a consultant and have the procedure to remove the damaged parathyroid gland(s).

I was one of the lucky ones as, even though I was undiagnosed for a couple of years, my GP referred me to an endocrinologist as they were curious as to 'why my blood calcium levels were slightly raised'. I did not have high calcium levels in my blood but was very unwell with every symptom listed for HPHT, with the exception of kidney problems. Unfortunately, I find myself dealing with kidney issues post operation which I believe to be a result of having higher calcium levels in my body for a couple of years, pre diagnosis.

So many people suffering with this condition can go undiagnosed for years as many GPs are unfamiliar with PHPT (my own GP had to Google it!) and do not see slightly raised levels of calcium as a reason for referring a patient onto a specialist. My main reason for writing, is to highlight the many cases of those who are not as fortunate as me. By ignoring or being ignorant of this disease, there are large numbers of people who are suffering with a life altering condition and who, unlike me, will not be fortunate enough to have a curious GP. For this reason, I would urge you to consider recognition of PHPT in its different classifications and ask if the harm caused to many by medical ignorance, can be justified. Thank you for your time.

Yours sincerely

Jane Church (nee Coles)

Jay

I write in support of letter **reference SJP/SS-CEONHS/15-03-21** and to highlight my individual primary hyperparathyroid (PHPT) journey, associated difficulties encountered along the way and requests for action.

I became unwell around 2017, with incrementally but noticeably worsening symptoms until the present day. Following an initial (minor) swimming injury to my knee in February 2019, from which I still have not fully recovered, MSK investigations identified deficient vitamin D, the second 50,000 iu dose of which resulted in a seven and a half hour admission to A&E and my PHPT diagnosis.

During the six months post-swimming injury, I visited my GP increasingly regularly, with growing concern about pains, feared damage to my back or knee, and simply very odd occurrences with my body. By the end of June 2019, I was sometimes visiting my GP twice a week, to be told that all my symptoms were in my head and that, if I continued to visit her, she would 'do something about my mental health'.

This GP-level gas-lighting and lack of awareness is my first **request for action**. My GP at the time did not conduct a calcium or PTH test, simply prescribing Vit D. Moreover, she would not have requested even the Vit D bloods if it were not for my very persistent MSK team.

During my visit to A&E on 30 June, 2019, an excellent team did test my calcium and suggested that I revisit matters with my GP. This I did, taking a full and detailed written summary of my symptoms from January 2019 to July 2019, along with a comparative 'then and now' set of photos, since by this point it was apparent that I clearly even looked like a very different person.

Once again, I was dismissed and ridiculed, and it was suggested that I see another GP since she 'could no longer deal with me'. Eventually, following a thirty-minute discussion and supported by a good friend, this GP very reluctantly agreed to test PTH and calcium. Three days later, the same GP rang to give me my very conclusive blood results and, without apology, told me over the phone that I had PHPT. I have changed my GP to another within the same practice, but even this GP had told me that I now know more than she does about PHPT. The **action** that I am requesting is strengthening of the current GP/medical school training, the provision of additional resources to GP practices and the communication of clear guidelines to GPs.

Following my diagnosis in July 2019, I then paid privately to ensure that I was not left in a queue to see an endocrinologist for onwards referral to a surgeon, as a result of which I started the series of standard PHPT tests under the team at St James in Leeds. I live in Calderdale, which is a good hour's drive from Leeds, but asked for this referral as the team in Calderdale do not undertake sufficient parathyroidectomies (50 per annum) to be deemed expert in what is actually a complex illness.

This brings me to my second request for **action**, which is that regional centres of excellence be created for the treatment of PHPT, rather than leaving this to individuals to identify and resource themselves. This should be at the level of the region, with individuals being able to reach a centre of excellence within a one and a half hour drive. Such centres should have experienced and highly trained surgeons and, most importantly, scan facilities and staff.

I have relatively high PTH (around 25), high adjusted calcium (2.77) and stubbornly deficient Vit D, despite continuous and ongoing supplementation. I was operated on in July 2020, unsuccessfully. I had three experienced surgeons in my neck for 2.5 hours of what was a 4 hours 45 minutes operation, but my adenoma is ectopic and was not found during that surgery. I was told by the (experienced?) team there, that if their last available scan – a 4D CT – did not locate my adenoma, I would simply be referred back to their endocrinologists, as there was nothing more they would do, and that no surgeon would offer any further surgery in the absence of localisation.

This is my third request for **action**, that these specialist centres should themselves be updated on best practice relating to the care of those of us with ectopic glands. As I discovered with the support of Hyperparathyroid UK Action4Change, there is more that can and should be done, including further scans of a more specialist nature.

I was in the fortunate position being able to fund a private consultation and to make a request to be transferred to the care of Professor Palazzo in London, under whose team I am now awaiting a more sophisticated scan.

However, I live some 250 miles away from London and it is virtually impossible to make this journey in Covid times. Moreover, given my deteriorated physical health, this journey will be a difficult one even in a more normal world, which leads me to my fourth request for **action** around resources. PHPT patients with ectopic glands should not be subject to a postcode lottery; we should have the more specialist scans (that is the Choline/PET scan) available at a regional level. Moreover, those of us with enduring and persistent disease post-first op should be supported by inclusion on, for example, the JVCI list of illnesses and free prescription eligibility; in my case, for example, if I do not supplement my Vitamin D that would lead to emergency A&E admission as my levels are very low (DESPITE initial boosts and 2,000 iu), yet I have no financial support for this and am not on the JVCI vaccination lists, presumably because this is a rare position and a rare illness, largely affecting menopausal women who are not heard.

Funding of some of these requested actions would be through large savings if those of us with PHPT received correct diagnosis and treatment in a timely manner. For example, in my case, I have had several visits to A&E and PenDoc; MRI; 6 months of physio; a 24-hour ECG; MSK referral for 4 months; and approximately 7 hours' (in hindsight) unnecessary GP surgery hours pre-diagnosis.

To summarise, the requested actions here and in **SJP/SS-CEONHS/15-03-21** are:

- Updated NICE guidelines;

- Dedicated specialist PHPT teams, including a dedicated PHPT endocrinologist within each Trust and specialist regional surgical centres of excellence;

- Enhanced and refreshed GP training, with updated supporting web-based materials for both patients and GPs;

- A change to the current postcode lottery system for those with PHPT, with improved resources (notably scanning staff and facilities) within daily commute distance across the UK.

Kind regards,

Jay

A copy of this letter has also been sent to Professor Amanda Howe, President of RCGP.

<u>J H</u>

Dear Sir Stevens

Re: Campaign for radical improvement in understanding, recognition and treatment of Primary Hyperparathyroidism

Reference: Hyperparathyroid UK letter SJP/SS-CEONHS/15-3-21

I am writing to support the above letter instigated by the Hyperparathyroid UK Action4Change group, and would like to share my story to enable you to understand the difficulties people face in order to achieve a satisfactory, timely diagnosis and treatment for Hyperparathyroidism. From this group I have gained a wealth of knowledge and support, enabling my better understanding of the condition, of which I had no previous awareness.

In January 2020 I had a routine over fifties health check which revealed high blood calcium of 2.85mmol/L (normal range 2.2 - 2.6). Additional testing showed parathyroid hormone (PTH) level of 11.3pmol/L (normal range 1.6 – 6.9).

I was subsequently referred to the Mineral Metabolism Clinic for 24-hour urine collection which showed high calcium levels. A DEXA bone density scan revealed osteoporosis in my lumber spine -2.5 and osteopenia in my right hip, I am 56 years of age. These results confirmed a diagnosis of Primary Hyperparathyroidism in September 2020. I was referred for surgery, and on the recommendation of the Hyperparathyroid UK Action4Change group, I contacted Mr Shad Khan at Oxford University Hospital for treatment. Mr Khan is an exceptional, well-respected surgeon who I believe performed ninety five parathyroid operations last year in addition to 150 other endocrine surgeries.

I had a relatively straightforward operation on 16 January 2021 when my pre-op blood calcium level was 2.92. For years I had been feeling increasingly unwell, with a great deal of pain in my bones and joints, extreme fatigue, memory problems, difficulty in concentrating, excessive thirst, blurred vision and the feeling that the joy of life had deserted me, to name a few of my symptoms. These have had a detrimental effect on my working life as well as my family and personal life.

On reviewing my medical records, I note that in July 2014 I had raised calcium levels of 2.64 having visited my GP with symptoms which I now recognise as being in line with Hyperparathyroidism, however no further action was taken. I subsequently visited my GP in September 2016, again concerned that I was still suffering from these symptoms. However, it was assumed that these were symptoms of the menopause and although I was prescribed HRT to deal with the hot flushes I was experiencing, many other symptoms persisted.

I believe there were missed opportunities for an early diagnosis of primary hyperparathyroidism, and more timely treatment could have prevented the onset of osteoporosis in my spine and the damage which the very high levels of calcium in my blood have had to every organ in my body

I propose that better understanding of the symptoms and serious health implications of primary hyperparathyroidism needs to be urgently recognised by members of the medical profession. This would result in significant savings to the NHS, and the improvement in the lives of the many women and men who are affected by it. The NICE guidelines are outdated and need to be rewritten in line with recent research.

I was fortunate that a routine health check picked up the high calcium levels in my blood, I received a relatively swift diagnosis and successful surgery resulted in the removal of an 18mm adenoma, meaning I am now cured of this insidious disease. However, my recovery has been slow, I believe that as I have been suffering from this disease since at least 2014, a significant amount of damage has been wreaked on my body since then. Others have not been so fortunate and have struggled for many years to achieve a basic level of understanding and compassion leading to a successful diagnosis and ultimately surgery.

There is only one cure for primary hyperparathyroidism, and that is surgery in the hands of an experienced surgeon. I would urge you to contact Mr Shad Khan Shahab.khan@ouh.nhs.uk who can further explain the implications of this disease and how timely diagnosis and surgery can save the NHS valuable time and resources.

Yours sincerely

J H

Jayne

Jayne lives in Western Australia. This is a letter she wrote to her endocrinologist to raise awareness, which she forwarded to Simon Stevens;

Normocalcemic Primary Hyperparathyroidism

I was glad to see that an online GP Education event on Parathyroid disease was held at the end of March 2020, and therefore felt it was an opportune time to contribute to greater understanding of the disease by adding my scenarios below.

As a former parathyroid patient and registered nurse, I felt it important to send an update on the outcome of my second episode of hyperparathyroidism; 'Normocalcemic' primary hyperparathyroidism.

First Operation

Prior to my first parathyroid surgery in 2012, in previous years since 2009, I had been hospitalised and treated for major depression and kidney stones before finally calcium and parathyroid hormone blood levels were tested and primary hyperparathyroidism was diagnosed.

Subsequently, in various forums, I have found that many patients across the world suffer this unnecessary experience.

Blood tests taken in February 2012 prior to my first operation showed Calcium 2.96, Corrected; 2.82 (2.1-2.6), parathyroid hormone 15 (0.7-7.0), and Vitamin D 57 (>50)

My first parathyroid surgery in 2012 removed a large 750mg parathyroid adenoma that was seen on a sestamibi contrast scan but no other parathyroid glands were checked. The following case outcome indicates, I believe, that further education is advisable, and will be helpful for patients in the future.

Normocalcemic confusion

Hyperparathyroidism symptoms unfortunately returned from 2015 onwards with mid normal calcium levels and high normal to abnormal parathyroid hormone levels in the following years. I was diagnosed with fibromyalgia and IBS at this time in 2016. I had seen you previously, and you diagnosed my Primary Hyperparathyroidism in 2012.

Despite this, Primary Hyperparathyroidism symptoms continued to increase. My GP referred me for a 4D CT nuclear medicine scan in 2017. It reported new Thyroid cysts and a possible parathyroid adenoma on the right side.

I returned to see the previous endocrine surgeon who sent me to have the thyroid cysts biopsied but dismissed the parathyroid symptoms because blood levels were not clinically the classic primary hyperparathyroidism abnormal levels.

2nd Operation

A new surgeon gave a second opinion and monitored me for six months. Metabolic bone study, blood and urine tests in June 2018 showed abnormally high urine calcium levels: 74umol/L GF (9-42) and urine calcium/creatinine 1.13mol/L (0.10-0.58)

A repeat bone density scan showed worsening osteoporosis; from moderate to severe, between 2016 and 2018.

Blood tests in August 2017 reported calcium 2.23, Corr. 2.31 (2.1-2.55); parathyroid hormone 7.3, (1.6-6.9) and Vitamin D 65 (51-150). Blood tests in June 2018 reported calcium 2.38, Corr. 2.28; parathyroid hormone 6.6, and Vitamin D 68.

As a result of those findings, a second parathyroid surgery was arranged in June 2018; an exploratory surgery of the right side, by the surgeon. A 90mg Parathyroid adenoma was removed and a biopsy of the other parathyroid gland on the same side showed no hyperplasia.

Learnings from second operation

Calcium, parathyroid hormone and Vitamin D levels should be tested at the same time, and several tests graphed to see how they are trending, and to see if they are acting normally in relation to each other.

I feel it is important to make GP's and Doctors at all levels aware of this, so recurring symptoms are thoroughly investigated and are not dismissed or diagnosed as another condition. For example, in my case, I was incorrectly diagnosed with Fibromyalgia and IBS in 2016 when symptoms returned.

With my previous history of this disease, returned primary hyperparathyroidism symptoms, high normal to abnormal parathyroid hormone levels and a positive 4D CT scan indicating a possible parathyroid adenoma; these factors pointed to a parathyroid disease recurrence.

Post Operation

Post op my calcium levels dropped low as my Osteoporosis was and has been recovering and I now take calcium supplements to keep my calcium levels stable. I passed another small kidney stone in January 2019.

This year 2020, two years after my surgery my body systems are still recovering after having hyperparathyroid disease for such a long time.

Bone Density

My first Bone density scan was in 2016, four years after my first parathyroid surgery, which showed the osteoporosis was moderate. Parathyroidectomy post-operative care should also routinely include a bone density scan to monitor bone recovery.

Thankfully in August 2019 a bone density scan, one year after surgery, showed my osteoporosis had markedly improved to moderate osteoporosis in my spine, almost to osteopenia in my hip and slight improvement in the forearm.

Mental Health

Unfortunately I was being treated for symptoms only, during both primary hyperparathyroidism episodes, and the underlying medical problem was missed. I was treated for the mental health, kidney and digestive symptoms.

The traditional mnemonic for this condition is 'moans, groans, stones and bones'. Surely we should not have to wait till we have end organ involvement to get treatment as was my case this second episode.

I was hospitalised again with 'anxiety and depression' four months post-surgery which was later recognized as caused by Low calcium blood levels.

Ectopic heartbeats

I made three visits to ED with ectopic heartbeat episodes around six months post-surgery which was finally recognized as low calcium blood levels of 1.9 (2.1-2.6).

It was an afterhours GP who treated me by increasing my calcium supplements to 2.5G daily and gradually my calcium levels stabilized. I still have ectopic heartbeats whenever my calcium levels drop. I now take 1.2G calcium daily.

Information sources

I belong to the 'Hyperparathyroid UK Action4Change' support group, who have helped me to understand this disease. What I have learnt, backed by the UK NICE guidelines is that at least 5% of Primary Hyperparathyroid patients may not be successfully treated and have another parathyroid adenoma appear.

www.nice.org.uk/guidance/ng132

Normocalcemic Primary Hyperparathyroidism has been recognized in the UK since 2014.

During the second episode I had seventeen of the twenty one symptoms on the print out list from the Centre for Advanced Parathyroid Surgery in the USA; hyperparathyroidmd.com is Dr B. Larian's USA website that gives a thorough explanation of parathyroid disease and its different presentations.

Dr Larian and his team perform 4000 Parathyroidectomy surgeries a year, so see a large group of patients and can be considered an expert in this field. He gives his time without charge to answer questions from those of us having difficulty finding help with this often poorly recognized disease.

Conclusion

As a result of the long journey I have had with this disease, I am now recovering from osteoporosis, and resulting low calcium issues. It is known to develop over a long period and be asymptomatic for some time. I have probably had it developing since the late 1990's when I had surgery for very large ovarian cysts.

My hope in updating you of my case history is that parathyroid disease and its different presentations will be more recognized here in Perth. I am not alone in the difficulty of getting treatment the second time.

In this time of internet access to parathyroid disease, support groups and overseas specialists and surgeons for advice by patients, I feel doctors at all levels have the resources to be up to date as well.

Trusting you will take note of my concerns.

Yours faithfully,

Jayne

Jayne Wright

Dear Mr Stevens,

As someone with undiagnosed Primary Hyperparathyroidism (PHPT), for many years, I wanted to write to you to suggest some amendments to the 'NICE Guidelines' so that future sufferers are not prevented from having the essential treatment they urgently need.

My Calcium never went higher than 2.69mmol/L. Eventually, after many years of feeling unwell, in 2017, I actually had two adenomas removed privately, as the wait was too long on the NHS, with my levels, not really deemed high enough. Fortunately my husband's company had private healthcare so I didn't hesitate to push for an operation once I had persuaded a Dr to test PTH and Calcium from the same blood draw!

It shouldn't be like this. It's not rare. I have two close friends, a sister-in-law, a neighbour's son and a workman, all who needed surgery for this awful condition. The workman is still waiting!

My neighbour's son was told if he didn't have surgery soon he would need dialysis. It had been left so long, that shortly after he eventually had the op, he had a heart attack. Fortunately he survived, but it goes to exemplify the dangers of years of unchecked and untreated suffering from hyperparathyroidism.

From a heart scan, I too have calcifications, but I have never suffered from kidney stones. The range of symptoms which are so debilitating are varied and awful. PTH is not routinely screened so no one picked up what was wrong with me for years.

I had three painful calcific tendinitis operations on both shoulders unnecessarily, and I even asked to be checked for primary hyperparathyroidism when they were sucking out vials containing calcium from my shoulders (barbotage procedure). Sadly they only checked my calcium levels and decided I didn't have it without testing my PTH levels! Crazy!

Ironically, early diagnosis of primary hyperparathyroidism will save the NHS thousands of pounds. I have had several unnecessary operations and have seen several specialists (cardiologists, rheumatologists, orthopaedic surgeons) who all sadly missed a diagnosis of primary hyperparathyroidism. My calcium levels were never particularly high, so I was left until I diagnosed myself with PHPT following a blood test that revealed low Vitamin D levels. As I supplemented vitamin D, I felt even more terrible.

I searched online in desperation and found parathyroid.com which saved my life. I then found Hyperparathyroid UK Action4Change Facebook group. I have read about hundreds of similar battles, really unwell people have had to fight, simply trying to get diagnosed and surgery, from poorly informed GPs and endocrinologists. At their lowest ebb, these folks are trying to persuade GPs and consultants to take their needs seriously, whilst they are told to adopt a 'watch and wait' approach. It is a slow death...it feels dreadful!

I can't change what happened to me but I can make the case to persuade you to make an NHS change that will actually be cost effective and ensure people's lives are not made a misery, and endangered by this 'watch and wait' approach. I implore you to reconsider training doctors, and amending NICE guidelines, to ensure others do not suffer daily from the ongoing pain and issues that I have, because early diagnosis was denied. It is not menopause, stress, ME, fibromyalgia, or simply a lack of vitamins, or anaemia...the list of excuses goes on. Anyone with kidney issues, heart issues and generalised exhaustion with aches and pains or mental ill health issues should be routinely screened with a blood test for Ca/PTH and Vitamin D. Simple!

I recognise the timing of this request is tricky due to COVID and I want to pay tribute to the amazing work currently happening to support COVID patients, but equally this situation cannot be ignored and is hurting thousands of people. I look forward to hearing from you that systemic change is going to become a reality. Please read Sallie's letter - her words sum it up very well.

Yours faithfully

Jayne

Kath Yates

Dear Sir Simon Stevens

From around 1987/88 I suffered for ten years plus, with extreme tiredness. My days consisted of getting my two girls off to school and spending the rest of the day having my house ship shape, shopping and having meals ready for husband and girls returning home.

To do this my timetable consisted of getting my jobs done, but in between, having to rest numerous times to build up my energy. During these years of suffering I visited my GP on many occasions, always to be told my blood tests were fine. I somehow could never get through to them that my tiredness wasn't just the everyday tiredness. I just needed to keep resting and didn't feel right. In later years I started to get very bad bone pain in my elbows, more visits to GP but still no further progress.

By 2011/12. I had bone pain in my hands, legs and feet and was also suffering from brain fog. I couldn't concentrate, was very forgetful. These symptoms and the brain fog were getting me down, I even gave up driving as I didn't feel safe.

Around August/September 2012, I went to my GP to say my symptoms were getting me down and I couldn't cope. I had a blood test and when the results came back my GP said 'There is something'. The Calcium in my blood was very high. I was referred to Endocrinologist, had various tests, and was told not to worry as they would make me feel better.

On 5th January 2013 I had one parathyroid adenoma removed from the right side of my neck. **Two days into my recovery my brain fog had disappeared and I felt like I was back on earth.** I felt a new woman with more energy and my bone pain was disappearing. I was discharged a few months later and the last thing the surgeon said to me was, "just remember it can return."

At this time my husband was suffering kidney failure and was on dialysis. He would eventually need a transplant. I had to wait 2 years to get over my parathyroidectomy before I could be tested for a

Kidney donor. He went on the waiting list. After 2yrs I was tested and was a match. On 8th March 2016 my spare kidney was donated and successfully transplanted and all was fine.

By 2019 I started again with bone pain, fatigue, brain fog and numbness in my feet and I remembered the surgeon saying my hyperparathyroidism could come back. So, back I went to GP for a blood test. He told me my calcium was fine. After a few visits and still being told Calcium was fine and also being told my problem was I was depressed, I said otherwise, as I was also getting breathless on incline.

Since then I have been put on Steroids. I've had my heart checked, stamina tested on a treadmill and had numerous CT scans, x-rays etc., but I still wonder if I have another adenoma as I have all the same symptoms and more. The trouble is, since I joined this site of Hyperparathyroid UK, with Sallie Powell, who has been a God send to lots of poorly people, it has come to light that lots of endocrinologist don't follow the correct NICE guidelines and the correct procedure for a good outcome.

We, on the Hyperparathryoid UK site, hope that by trying to increase awareness by good people like yourself, we can make a change and help stop people suffering from this terrible disease and give Sallie Powell the recommendation she deserves.

Thank you for your attention

Kath Yates.

Kathy Sassoon

Dear Sir or Madam,

I am writing to you as a member of Hyperparathyroid UK Action4Change. After the last few years of listening to hundreds of people like myself struggle with getting diagnosis for a simple endocrine disease that cuts a swathe of disability through otherwise highly productive lives, it's now time for us all to start acting.

In 2019 we had high hopes for the NICE guidelines on PHPT which turned out to change very little in reality.

I was a "lucky" patient in the end who had such high levels of calcium and parathyroid and was ten days from diagnosis to surgery thanks to private insurance. However I had such severe re-mineralising symptoms post operatively that I was bedbound again for nearly a year and had no guidance or acceptance from any medical practitioner let alone any help. If it hadn't been for Sallie Powell's Facebook page and her personal knowledge, I would still be seriously ill nearly five years on.

It is not acceptable that we have to use collective knowledge through social media to understand our medical condition because the medical protocols are not fit for purpose. In my experience, the use of "normal range" diagnosis means that the endocrine suppressive relationship between calcium and parathyroid hormone is misunderstood and misdiagnosed daily. It is easy for GPs and endocrinologists to follow the current tick box process but unfortunately this keeps a huge number of very ill people in the way of continuing harm.

Surely people who have successfully completed a medical degree and specialist training could be trained a bit more deeply about this condition which is the third most common endocrine disease in the UK, the least understood and poorly diagnosed.

The only people who do understand the situation and are attempting to educate more widely are a small clutch of intellectually curious and experienced parathyroid surgeons who see our concerns proven as a result of their work, that things are very seriously amiss.

Patients, middle aged women in particular, are being basically abused by medical personnel by constant misdiagnosis and disbelief at the global nature of these symptoms. Abuse is a big word to use but it has really come to this. No middle aged woman or man has any desire to continually push to get medical attention without due cause.

I live in Western Australia and am pleading for some attention to this issue. Our health system follows the UK and any light that can be shed will have benefits for us too. In our state anyone without absolutely clear classic presentation of this condition has no chance of diagnosis or treatment, and most cases of high calcium are passed off as secondary due to vitamin D deficiency, which isn't shown by blood tests or 'genetic' with no tests performed to back it up.

There are no effective protocols to guide GPs or pathology labs to pick this up for patients. Recently most pathology labs have extended the normal range for parathyroid hormone from (1.6-6.9) to (1.6-9) for the stated reason of avoiding negative scans, as they cost too much.

The issue here is that diagnosis is by blood test, not by scan which should be used only by surgeons for location purposes. Shifting scans into aids for diagnosis has resulted in this cost cutting measure. It is already having the impact of removing diagnosis for a whole raft of patients who now have to wait years, possibly decades for their levels to reach extreme heights, risking end organ damage and the destruction of their marital, work and social lives for a protocol change that has no actual medical basis to it.

The money and time that could be saved for medical services by attending to this correctly is immense, not to mention the intense, life changing suffering that would be relieved for so many.

We are asking for some serious attention to this for the benefit of the thousands of patients currently leading unproductive lives for no reason. A review of the NICE protocols in consultation with Sallie Powell and the surgeons who really understand this condition in all classifications. A commissioning of the appropriate research into primary hyperparathyroidism is urgently required. Thank you so much for your attention.

Yours faithfully,

Kathy Sassoon

kathy@leucacreek.com.au

June Blunden

Our Ref. SJP/SS-CEO/NHS/ 15-3-21

Dear Sir Simon Steven,

Can I please draw your attention to the difficulty people with the disease Primary Hyper parathyroidism have in getting diagnosis?

I have suffered with primary hyperparathyroidism for many years longer than needed, simply because the people that I consulted about my symptoms didn't have the necessary information to correctly diagnose me.

Consequently it was left to my GP over time to refer me to several unnecessary consultants for investigation into the many symptoms I had. This resulted in wasted NHS resources both in consultants' time and the many procedures I had, all of which were not needed.

Between 2003 and 2009 I had a very poor quality of life until eventually being offered two scans on the area of the glands. Both showed abnormalities. At this point I was offered an operation which was carried out in 2010 and proved successful.

Sadly, in 2013 I Once again began to have symptoms. However, I was once again turned away by the endocrinologist who repeated his previous decision, that my blood calcium levels were not high enough to diagnose a problem with my parathyroid glands.

I was devastated as I knew he was wrong. At this point I was left with no choice but to pay for a private consultation with a consultant who I was advised had more knowledge of the decease.

After the necessary scans and procedures I had a further operation. In total the cost to me was £9700. This was money I could not afford and I feel thoroughly let down by the NHS.

In conclusion I hope you will look into the reason why staff working within the service appear to have a lack of the knowledge, which is available to them and as a consequence are causing many thousands of pounds of wasted NHS funds.

Yours sincerely,

June Blunden

Kim Cox

THIS IS MY STORY

Another start to another week in this half-life that I have been living for as long as I can remember. Am I the only person who is dreading Lockdown ending? I haven't got the energy to face 'normal life' again – it will mean travelling, mixing with lots of other people and trying to cope with entire days instead of these half days I exist in.

It is now two years, eleven months and fourteen days since I had to step down from my four day a week management position which I had enjoyed for seven years previously, to struggling to work two full days a week, and am currently working three afternoons so that I don't have to wonder if the morning is going to be average or hell, and the pressure of whether I can make it or not.

The cause of this loss of my career and life, is primary hyperparathyroidism, which was diagnosed in the summer of 2019, although I had been feeling unwell for some time before – hence the need to cut my working time. I was so ill that I actually went to my manager to tell her I needed to resign as I no longer had the energy to do the job I so loved. Fortunately she was so switched on that she suggested cutting my hours and staying to do the parts of the job that were my favourite. As she put it 'You don't want to be at home all the time – you need to get out and have a bit of a challenge'. Thank goodness she did persuade me to stay on. otherwise this situation would be worse than ever.

So, my diagnosis came as such a relief, and my doctor immediately booked me an appointment with the endocrinologist at our local hospital for about five weeks later, July 2019. I was so excited that at last it had a name and 'they' were going to put it right.

The appointment was cancelled and that doctor left the surgery to live elsewhere. Another appointment was given – this time in October 2019. Also cancelled. I never received another appointment letter and just limped on.

Covid came, and with it of course came the 'Barrier' to all other medical care. No endocrinology appointment, impossible to see a doctor, and feeling under par most of the time.

It was towards the end of the first Lockdown that I started to feel worse – instead of having one or sometimes two 'good' days a week, I woke up feeling dreadful every morning.

No matter how much sleep I have, I wake up with shoulder pain, headaches, dizziness, nausea, pains in my ankles, knees and elbows and often low mood. Some days are like walking through treacle, and the brain fog that is so frequent, makes it hard to get motivated. I can't even read a magazine – let alone a book.

Between lockdowns, I managed to see another GP, who tested my appropriate blood levels and confirmed my diagnosis. When the bloods came back, I was advised to 'drink more water'. After a day or two pondering this, I rang the surgery and queried how much is 'more' when they don't even know what I normally drink.

After the second GP - who just kept reminding me that I would be low priority as my calcium level was only just above the borderline, so it would be considered that it wasn't severe - passed me onto the third GP – who called me 'an enigma'.

I eventually managed to see a fourth GP in the practice who took a positive view and I asked for a direct referral to Mr Shad Khan, an endocrine surgeon at Oxford University Hospitals.

However, she explained I would have to have the operation in Wales as I live in Wales. She managed to get me a cancellation with endocrinology at the hospital. I thought that my worries were over and at long last the endocrinologist would refer me to a surgeon in Wales – WRONG!

It is now a month since I saw him for the first time. This year is the first time I have had the requisite Vitamin D blood test, along with calcium and PTH. He has taken two sets of Bloods and decided to put me on a high dose of Vitamin D (Fultium D 800iu x 4 a day) to see if it's a Vitamin D deficiency. I feel no better and he seems to be against operations for primary hyperparathyroidism for various reasons. I will be seeing him again in April. What will happen then goodness knows…………………………………………

Yours sincerely

Kim D Cox

Lesley Craig

Professor Amanda Howe
President RCGP

Our Ref: SJP/AH-RCGP/15-03-21

My problems with GP on my journey to get diagnosed with Hyperparathyroidism

I had a scan which confirmed an adenoma in December 2019 - the endocrinologist who was monitoring my Neuro Endocrine Tumour had arranged for this after I had described my PHPT symptoms - these previously dismissed by GP for three years.

The endocrinologist then sent through a letter to my GP proposing a referral to a local experienced surgeon in January 2020. This was not actioned by my GP until I raised the issue in September 2020 - I guess Covid taking priority in everyone's minds which is understood.

I was surprised that the GP commented that I "obviously had an itch I needed to scratch" before agreeing to send the recommended referral. I found this comment both unnecessary and patronising. It also seemed so out of character and has left me with a very negative impression.

I'm glad to say from that point I've been seen, listened to, and an operation for removal of the parathyroid adenoma has been agreed - just waiting for Covid to release its grip before a date can be arranged.

I think the experience I've had highlights the importance of having to be pro-active with all medical professionals and not rely on assuming they are on top of everything.

GP's essentially are the gatekeepers for any NHS treatment - if they are ignorant or ill-informed (about certain conditions), closed minded and biased, patients are left to languish unless they can afford private care or are fortunate enough to join an action group. A GP's personal approach makes a vast difference to a patient's mental wellbeing as does being taken seriously. As an individual you feel totally powerless and angry in the hands of a dismissive and frequently unreachable GP.

With respect - what is the reputation you wish for as your legacy as President of RCGP's?

That GP's are highly valued and fully respected for their capabilities in medical practice,

Or

Are they to be viewed as distant, uncaring and only interested in making money - after all being a GP today is about managing finances - isn't it......?

Yours sincerely

Lesley Craig

Lesley Davidson

TO BE READ IN CONJUNCTION WITH LETTER FROM SALLIE POWELL

Dear Sir Simon Stevens

Action needed by NHS England for recognition and treatment of Hyperparathyroidism

MY POSITIVE JOURNEY OF HOW NORMOCALCAEMIC HYPERPARATHYROIDISM SHOULD BE TREATED

Please make time to read and digest my positive journey regarding my **normocalcaemic primary hyperparathyroidism** and its diagnosis. I consider myself to be extremely lucky. Sadly, this is not happening with a huge majority of cases.

DIAGNOSIS HISTORY

October – December 2019
- Over a very short period of time I began to feel both physical and mentally unwell, nothing you could put your finger on but my whole demeanour changed. I was normally a physically active person (for my age, 64), trim, ate a healthy diet and had a very positive attitude on Life. I continued going downhill and by December decided I needed to see a GP.

January 2019
- I visited my wonderful GP (he had known me for over 15 years), he listened, completely understood, was proactive and organised several lots of blood tests. **On each occasion my blood test results showed as 'normal' i.e. within range**.
- On the third visit to my surgery, I saw a new young GP. She had never seen me before. She listened whilst I went through my symptoms, which were steadily worsening. She had seen my previous blood results and thought there might be a chance I had a problem with my parathyroid glands. I had never heard of them, she explained their function etc. More bloods taken. In the meantime, she referred me to the endocrinology team at Weston

super Mare Hospital, North Somerset (my then nearest hospital). I must admit (shamefully) that I really had no confidence in the GP.

February 2019
- More blood tests done and yet again they all came back within range. The new GP said she was almost certain that I had parathyroid problems.

March 2019
- Phone call from my usual GP to have a chat about my pre-existing lung condition. I mentioned that my endocrinology appointment was the next day, and that I didn't know how to prepare for it. He said he didn't think it would come to anything, neither did I.
- **Initial endocrinology appointment**: I was asked to describe my symptoms. I enlightened the specialist to the fact that I didn't actually know what he was looking for. He went through many possible symptoms **including the ones I had; depression, tiredness, feeling continually thirsty, feeling sick, muscle weakness, muscle/bone pain, word 'blindness', stomach pains, lack of concentration**. After fully explaining verbally and showing screen shots of diagrams of parathyroid glands I began to fully understand the condition that he was sure I had; he was almost 100% certain that I had normocalcaemic primary hyperparathyroidism (NCPHPT) and would need surgery. He would make a referral to Southmead Hospital, Bristol, as they had a very knowledgeable team in NCPHPT. My referral was marked 'urgent' as I was going downhill so rapidly.

May – August 2019
- Three further appointments with endo team to monitor me. Full bloods taken after each appointment, all results came back within range apart from latterly when the parathyroid hormone (PTH) result was higher. **My highest adjusted calcium was 2.65!**

September 2019
- I had an initial appointment with a surgeon, Justin Morgan (privately due to my imminent house move from Somerset to Cornwall), accompanied by my husband who was there to make a mental note of what Mr Morgan said. By this stage my memory was terrible. Mr Morgan listened as I went through my symptoms and without looking at any of my blood test results agreed that I

was presenting with NCPHPT and would require surgery. He explained that without surgery my bone strength would definitely deteriorate, resulting in osteopenia and osteoporosis. A specialist ultra sound scan (USS) and a vocal chord check would be organised with a view to surgery. The USS would, hopefully, detect where the glands were as unlike other organs in the body, they could be ectopic. The vocal chord check was to make sure that everything was in order.

- Mr Morgan fully explained NCPHPT to me, adding that it was a newly acknowledged condition. He added that if I had gone to a neighbouring hospital my operation would not have been considered as many surgeons do not 'recognise' it/refuse to acknowledge it!
  - **He recommended I join the Facebook group Hyperparathryoid UK Action4Change**, it was run by several very knowledgeable people and was a very friendly group.

October 2019

- USS scan undertaken. Three glands located, all enlarged, one particularly big.
- Vocal chord check. All in order.
- 25 October I have a three gland parathyroidectomy. The fourth gland was discovered during surgery. Mr Morgan did a four gland investigation and tagged the remaining gland with titanium in case it needed to be extracted in the future.
- 26 October I was discharged from hospital. I have hyperplasia. Hopefully the remaining gland should serve me well for the rest of my life. I was told about aftercare, self-care, remineralisation, hungry bone syndrome, and given calcium/vitamin D, which I continue to take.

Post op

- I felt an immediate improvement in my health, the brain fog went instantly together with the headaches, bone and muscle pain. I gradually recovered and became myself again.
- I had occasion to see my normal GP and mentioned NCPHPT. He admitted that he had never heard of it. I emailed him all the information that I had and requested that he disseminate the information to all the staff. Hopefully he did.

OBSERVATIONS

- By chance I saw a newly qualified GP who had been trained in Bristol. She knew about all aspects of hyperparathyroidism.
- Southmead Hospital (Bristol NHS) are held in very high regard regarding this condition and seem to be working towards being a centre of excellence.
- Weston Super Mare Endocrinology Department (Bristol NHS) work in tandem with Southmead Hospital.
- If you have three tiers (GP, endo, and surgeon) all knowledgeable and working as a complete team – the result can be remarkable.

I finish by saying that everyone deserves to receive the exceptional level of care, respect and consideration that I received.
Unfortunately, this is not the case in the vast majority of cases.

You can make a change for the positive. Please do it. Now.

Yours sincerely

Lesley Davidson

LH 1

Ref: SJP/AH-RCGP/15-3-21

Dear Professor Howe

Further to Sallie J Powell's letter to you, reference above, concerning Primary Hyperparathyroidism, which I totally and wholeheartedly support, I am writing to advise you of the awful and neglectful treatment that my husband experienced by two GP's from our practice following being diagnosed with Phpt.

My husband had been referred to a consultant endocrinologist by his gastroenterologist as his calcium level was raised. The appointment was 23rd October 2017. Following further blood tests on 25th October where his Calcium level had increased higher still, a diagnosis of Phpt was made and scans ordered. Unfortunately, neither us, nor the GP had been sent the letter advising any of this. I chased that letter from 6th November and was eventually contacted by telephone on the 5th December. The content of the letter was read out to me and posted first class. I requested that our GP was sent it ASAP. I advised that my husband had been getting worse during the weeks of not knowing anything or receiving any communication and that I was worried and asked if his Endocrinologist could please ring me. He didn't.

The next day 6th December, my husband was much worse so I made him an appointment with one of our GP's. I advised him of his Phpt diagnosis and that we had only received that information yesterday, as the surgery had too. I explained how poorly he feels and the symptoms he had; thirst, weight loss, nausea, loss of appetite, and constipation. How he kept losing his ability to concentrate, then his short term memory was affected, it got worse and he was very fatigued, he could no longer read or operate his computer. Our GP's response to our request for help was, he's under an Endocrinologist so not getting involved in that. I asked him to look at him and said he needs help. He prescribed antidepressant drugs! I also advised that I was worried about his diabetes and asked if giving him Nutri Bullet fresh fruit drinks was ok, he confirmed it was but didn't test his level, and he didn't examine him at all.

The next time I asked a GP for help was on 18th December after emailing the endocrinologist for help as I was so concerned about my husband and what was happening to him, his reply was contact your GP it's their responsibility!

Quite how that was the case when he was under that Endocrinologist's care I do not know. In fact when I had previously contacted him for help on 11th December, he called me on the 12th December, ordered blood tests and prescribed Cinacalcet as my husband was so poorly. I can't understand what was different on 18th.

I contacted our surgery immediately after reading his reply and requested an urgent home visit. The GP on Call rang me. I advised her of my husband's Phpt diagnosis, explained my concerns about my husband's deteriorating health, and told her I was extremely worried for him. Her response was, she was on the computer and doing something involving the NHS online and that she would come in the morning. She should have known the importance of responding quickly with a patient displaying his symptoms and with a diagnosis of Phpt. When she hadn't come by 12 the next day I contacted the surgery again.

She rang back and started asking the same questions that I had answered the afternoon before. When she came she could see how very poorly he was. I explained again the importance of testing his Calcium level, she left saying she would send the request to Phlebotomy as soon as she got back to her office. I spoke to her again the next afternoon on 19th December when still no one had been. By early afternoon on 20th December I was too worried to wait any longer and telephoned Phlebotomy to enquire when they were coming as I was so very concerned. They quickly confirmed that no request had been received for my husband. We both contacted the GP surgery who sent it to them immediately, advising that they had located it in my husband's notes and that the GP had forgotten to send it!
The manager in phlebotomy said she would come out herself and do his blood tests, which she did. On seeing how poorly he was, she advised she was taking them straight to the Lab.

Just after 5pm a GP rang, to advise that the Lab had just contacted him as my husband's Calcium level was 3.4 and that an ambulance was on the way to take him into hospital. The paramedics also identified high blood sugar 21.7 and tachycardia and he was seriously ill.

My husband was diagnosed with hypercalcemia secondary to Phpt and spent 15 days in hospital being treated. Having numerous intravenous infusions, as all of his electrolytes were out of balance and his health was seriously affect by this.

This should not have happened. My husband was under the care of a GP and an endocrinologist for a known diagnosed condition, both knew how ill he was, both should have had the knowledge required to effectively help him. I consider that both of them failed him.

A consultant, a so called specialist in this field, who doesn't think his patient's health is his responsibility, even though he is treating him and knows how poorly he is, having prescribed medication six days earlier.

An on-call GP that is too busy on line to respond to a very ill patient and when she does, she then forgets the most important task she had to do, send a simple request for a blood test. She also decided to ask a community psychiatrist for advice. It appeared to me that she didn't have any knowledge, understanding or experience of Phpt or she would have known that many Phpt patients suffer the same symptoms. It wasn't a psychiatrist he needed, it was surgery. She would also have known my husband was at risk of Hypercalcemia.

The other GP, in fact a senior partner, who didn't want to get involved and help my husband as he was under the care of an Endocrinologist, he didn't examine him, check his blood pressure or crucially get his calcium level tested or discuss anything with us, or test his blood sugar level, he just prescribed antidepressants. This senior GP should or would have known the risks and should have taken appropriate actions.

It is evident to me that many GP's and many other health professionals do not know enough about Phpt to effectively help and manage this illness. Whilst we can't expect them to have in depth knowledge about every illness, this is one of the most common Endocrine diseases that affects thousands of people. For many, including my husband, it's a life changing illness, affecting and damaging so many aspects of the body and sucks the joy from their lives.

In my husband's case he developed bilateral papilledema caused by high calcium and untreated Phpt, and required an urgent parathyroidectomy to save his sight. He remains in the care of ophthalmology as his peripheral sight is permanently damaged. He also developed heart arrhythmia and palpitations for which he requires prescription medication.

The only cure for Phpt is surgery and yet many GP's and endocrinologists apply a 'watch and wait' approach.
Wait for what? Osteoporosis, fractures, bone and joint problems, kidney stones, heart problems, depression, anxiety, cognitive and psychiatric problems, eye and teeth problems, the list goes on.

So many patients are misdiagnosed, fibromyalgia, depression and for many women it's the menopause.
Given many more women than men are affected, ratio is 3.1, and that many of them get it around the same time as the menopause, it is often undiagnosed for years. At what cost to the patient and to the NHS?

I speak with considerable knowledge of Phpt, having experienced the most horrendous management and treatment of my husband, undertaken significant research of Phpt and as a member of the Phpt Support Group, Hyperparathyroid UK Action4Change.

This group were responsible for campaigning for NICE Guidelines for Phpt and were key stakeholders in that process. Whilst they are not perfect and do require urgent revision and updating, we were excited and hopeful that things would improve for patients with this disease.

As a member of this group, I read daily posts and comments from other members about the difficulties in getting diagnosed, particularly by GP's, some of whom refuse to follow the Phpt guidelines, some don't even know there are guidelines. We had hoped and expected that publication of the guidelines would be notified to GP's through their updating mechanisms and arrangements. We hoped to see an improvement. Sadly, that is not the case. Many of our members have experienced years of misdiagnosis, being in a 'watch and wait' arrangement with damaging consequences as their health deteriorates. Some of their case stories are heart wrenching and all completely avoidable with the effective management of Phpt.

The NHS absolutely needs to raise awareness, early diagnosis is key, followed by surgery and good post-operative care, not just for the benefit of patients, who should and must be the priority here, but also importantly, to reduce the significant costs being incurred year upon year by the NHS.

Diagnosis of Phpt is for most patients straightforward and is easily cured by Parathyroidectomy surgery. Evidence shows that the cost of surgery is without doubt the most cost effective treatment.

If a parathyroidectomy had been performed following my husband's emergency admission with hypercalcemia, secondary to Phpt, the tragedy that unfolded would not have happened to him.

I ask most sincerely for your intervention and help to get this disease effectively recognised and managed within our NHS and very much hope that you will action the changes requested by Sallie J Powell for the benefit of patients and the NHS..

Yours sincerely

LH

LH 2

Ref: SJP/SS-CEO NHS/15-3-21

Dear Sir Simon Stevens,

Further to Sallie Powell's letter to you, referenced above, concerning primary hyperparathyroidism (PHPT), which I totally and wholeheartedly support, I am writing to advise you of the horrendous experiences my husband went through with PHPT, whilst under the care of NHS Doctors. Whilst I recognise this is a lot to read, I do urge you to read it, please. You need to know what many patients are up against through lack of training and essential knowledge of PHPT by Doctors. It is a hideous disease that sucks the joy out of your life. The impact this has on their quality of life, health, wellbeing, and that of their families can be shocking for some.

The costs associated with this disease not being well managed must be enormous due to misdiagnosis, 'watch and wait', progressive damage to bones, kidneys, heart, eyes, teeth, etc., when surgery will, in most cases cure the patient, avoid progressive illnesses and save significant amounts of money and resources. For example, I estimate that based on a cost of £400 per day, my husband's hospital admissions alone, all related to PHPT, cost the NHS £50,000, before the cost of involvement by five different specialisms, endocrinology, psychiatry, ophthalmology, neurology, and cardiology. Extremely excessive compared to the cost of a parathyroidectomy.

I am unsure exactly when my husband's raised calcium began. We suspect eighteen months before he was referred by a gastroenterologist to an endocrinologist in October 2017. The endocrinologist said calcium level of 2.63mmol/L, was not high, it was mild and he was going to discharge him. I raised concerns about his weight loss, muscle loss, and feeling unwell. Further blood tests a week later showed a significantly higher calcium level. Scans were arranged with a view to parathyroid surgery, having diagnosed primary hyperparathyroidism, although we were not made aware of this, but received two appointments for scans in November and December 2017.

I had been chasing a letter from the endocrinologist and was advised by telephone call on 5th December, that it hadn't been sent to us or to our GP. The content was read out to me, apologies were given and the letter was faxed to the GP and posted to us first class. I said I was extremely concerned about my husband and asked if the endocrinologist would please ring me, I did not receive a call back. Having been told he had Primary Hyperparathyroidism, I read up on the illness and symptoms, most of which he had, and I felt some relief that at last we knew what the problem was and he would have surgery and get well. I made contact again on 11th December, advising how ill my husband was, and again asked for his endocrinologist to please ring me. He telephoned the next day, organised a blood test form, and prescribed Cinacalcet 30 mg twice a day which my husband started taking that day, until his admission into hospital. His calcium continued to rise even though Cinacalcet was supposed to bring it down.

On the 18th of December he was so ill I emailed his endocrinologist as my husband was under his care. He told me it was the GP's responsibility and to contact them. I did so immediately but the GP would not visit until the following day. I rang the next day when she hadn't arrived by 12 pm. She arrived about an hour later. She said she would request blood tests on her return to the office. I spoke to her again the following afternoon 19th December, when a phlebotomist still hadn't been. At 1 pm on the 20th December, I was so worried, as my husband was deteriorating, I called phlebotomy myself, who confirmed they had not received anything from the GP. We both chased the GP surgery, who confirmed the GP had not sent the forms. They were sent immediately, blood taken, and urgently delivered to the lab around 3 pm that afternoon. Just after 5 pm, our GP phoned to say the lab had called as his calcium level was 3.4mmol/L, and that an ambulance was on its way to take my husband into hospital. The paramedics also identified high blood sugar at 21.7 and tachycardia. He was seriously ill. They phoned the hospital to warn of a medical emergency. We travelled under blue lights and sirens. I was so frightened for my husband and for his life. He was an emergency admission into hospital on 20th December 2017.

Resus was scary with doctors' quickly taking action to help him, literally running with blood samples. He went onto a ward during the night and continued to receive numerous intravenous infusions and treatments. Over 15 days, he was diagnosed with hypercalcemia secondary to PHPT. My husband was discharged from the hospital on 5th January 2018. They knew he was confused, yet offered him a mental health assessment and CT scan of his head, both of which were apparently refused. I wasn't advised of this until I saw it in the discharge summary. Given his confusion, which became much worse during his hospitalisation, I feel he was not in a position to make those choices. Where in this equation was any consideration or understanding of the mental health aspects of PHPT?

Our GP who saw him prior to his admission and following his discharge, stated very clearly that he should not have been discharged. The problem was a shortage of beds, and in my view, little or no knowledge of PHPT. The hospital advised that all of his electrolytes being out of balance, getting a UTI from a miss sited catheter, and low phosphate, can all cause confusion. His level of confusion had increased significantly during his stay.

Because so few doctors understand or have in-depth knowledge of PHPT, they try to treat the symptoms and not the cause. Sadly in my husband's case, no one seemed to understand the psychiatric problems that many PHPT patients suffer with, to varying degrees. Struggling to eat and drink due to nausea, loss of appetite and confusion, and feeling so ill, he was sectioned on 21st January 2019 and admitted into a mental health hospital. One of the psychiatrists involved in the section asked me my thoughts on why my husband was so confused and ill. I advised of my research on PHPT and explained the association with PHPT, psychiatric and cognitive problems that can occur. He replied that he thought I was most probably right.

This part of the journey had such an impact on me I began to have panic attacks. To this day I can't talk about what happened to my husband during this time without being extremely distressed. Writing this letter to you about what's happened has taken days and caused me distress.

Initially, he was prescribed sertraline and quetiapine. I had a meeting with his psychiatrist less than 24 hours after his admission, where she proceeded to talk about ECT and how she could legally decide whether to go ahead if she felt it necessary. I advised of my husband's position and views on ECT. I also tried to discuss his PHPT and how surgery is the only cure. She confirmed that she knew nothing about PHPT. I explained that many PHPT patients suffer from these problems. I requested her to do some research. I was horrified, and after that meeting, I sought urgent legal advice. Following that discussion with her, I wrote to her confirming my concerns and why imposing ECT would be against my husband's views and wishes. I also told her I would fight her if I needed to and would seek a second opinion. I was so worried about his health and him being forced down this mental health route instead of having the parathyroidectomy he so urgently needed, I requested his endocrinologist refer my husband to a professor of endocrinology, who he himself deferred to. His request and written communication from me were both ignored.

The drugs had little or no effect other than to cause falls, which I wasn't advised of. Against my wishes, Mirtazapine was added on 12th March. The impact on him was devastating. He was only able to shuffle a few steps, his head hung low, unable to communicate, lost and alone in a corridor, and now with incontinence.

I broke down the first time I found him like this. I requested an urgent meeting with his psychiatrist and insisted Mirtazapine was stopped and the others reduced. I questioned the benefits of these drugs, advising that some psychiatrists advise against prescribing these meds with PHPT and advise to treat the cause, not the symptoms. She openly admitted that she was treating the symptoms. I asked her if she had researched PHPT as I had requested at our first meeting. She said she had a telephone conversation with my husband's endocrinologist. Given that he felt out of his depth and had agreed to my request to refer my husband to an endocrine professor, I was very disappointed and unhappy, particularly as I had asked his endocrinologist to research the mental health aspects of PHPT. So their research consisted of just a telephone call to each other, the blind leading the blind. They were not listening or it appeared even caring.

At the beginning of April 2018, my husband's eyes were streaming with water, I asked a doctor to examine them. A trainee doctor on placement diagnosed dry eyes. My husband had several falls, one of which split his big toenail causing bleeding, pain, and soreness. I was advised that a chiropodist had been requested. When I enquired about it three days later, as no one had been, I was told it would be six weeks! Six weeks for an injury to be treated was completely unacceptable for any patient, let alone one with diabetes and a toe injury. I had no choice but to pay a private chiropodist, who was allowed in to treat him. Another fall resulted in a nasty head injury. He was taken to A&E by ambulance, and treated using steri strips where his forehead had split open. He was taken for an x-ray which I naturally assumed would be on his head but was on his chest. The steri strips were not stopping the blood and another doctor came to help. They applied more steri strips. I was left to get a wheelchair, get him to, and into the car, then drive him back to the mental health hospital. The on-call doctor was shocked he had not been kept in, as his head was still bleeding.

My husband's blood sugar became out of control; very low in the mornings 2.9 and 16/17 in the afternoon. It got so bad, yo-yo-ing from dangerously low to high that they were waking him about 6 am to test and give him juice and Weetabix to bring it up. His blood pressure also increased. Again I had to insist that advice was sought about his type two diabetes. I confirmed my concerns in writing. His medication was changed and his blood sugar levels improved and were back in range.

I had been led to believe that the MH hospital could meet my husband's physical and mental health needs, but that was not the case. The whole situation was like living in a nightmare. I had requested that his consultants work together, so parathyroid surgery could be progressed as this was the only cure. At an appointment with the surgeon in February 2018 he advised that the sestamibi scan was inconclusive and the ultrasound scan didn't show an adenoma but that a parathyroidectomy was needed, although cancer patients came first.

My husband was finally discharged from the MH hospital on 10th May 2018. Six days later, he attended his annual diabetic eye screening appointment. He was advised by letter that he had a swollen optic nerve in his left eye and had been urgently referred to the hospital eye clinic. Lots of eye scans and tests determined that both optic nerves were swollen and his sight damaged. The ophthalmologist advised they didn't know the cause and had urgently referred him to neurology.

At the appointment a few days later with a neurologist, he was admitted from the clinic to the neurology ward. An MRI the following day did not show any cause for the optic nerve swellings. As a result, they did a lumbar puncture, which also failed to identify a cause. My husband was diagnosed with bilateral papilledema, which I was told is both very serious and rare. He was referred to another hospital by post. I requested the referral be faxed which resulted in a telephone call that same afternoon, from an ophthalmologist surgeon who gave us an appointment two days later; 2nd July. We were there for hours for more eye scans, tests, and photographs. One of the two consultants asked why my husband had not had his surgery for PHPT. I explained all the events since 2017 and that his surgeon had said cancer patients come first. He replied that this surgery was just as urgent as cancer surgery. He confirmed that the cause of the swollen optic nerves was high calcium and untreated PHPT. He contacted the neurologist, advised the cause and that a parathyroidectomy was needed urgently to save his sight. My husband had an urgent parathyroidectomy surgery seven days later on 9th July 2018.

A three centimetre adenoma was removed. Initially, we were told by his surgeon that two 3cm adenomas had been removed, one lower left and one from his chest. This was revised following the histology report, discussed at the post-op appointment, to one 3cm lower left and parathyroid tissue from his chest. I understand that a three-centimetre adenoma is considered a whopper and would have been growing there for quite some time, to be that size.

My husband remains in the care of ophthalmology, with regular field view tests, eye tests, and monitoring, although currently delayed due to Covid risks as my husband is considered clinically extremely vulnerable. His peripheral sight is damaged, although following his parathyroid surgery there have been some improvements. My husband and I will forever be in debt to the consultant ophthalmologist surgeon who saved his sight and the ongoing progression of this insidious destructive disease that was destroying him.

Following my husband's discharge from the MH hospital, he was under the care of a consultant psychiatrist, who agreed his mental health problems were related to PHPT. He also advised that the medications were not helping, and both were withdrawn. He considered that my husband did not need any MH medication. He was discharged.

I am sure that you can't fail to see the significant consequences to my husband, caused by NHS Doctors with at best, poor, little or no understanding, knowledge, or experience of Phpt, resulting in unacceptable and inappropriate decisions, leading to significant damage to his health. My husband has arrhythmia problems, first caused by hypercalcemia and PHPT, and palpitations which is treated by prescription meds. If a parathyroidectomy had been performed following my husband's emergency admission with hypercalcemia secondary to Phpt, the tragedy that unfolded would not have happened to him.

I ask most sincerely for your intervention and help to get this disease effectively recognised and managed within our NHS and very much hope that you will action the changes requested by Sallie J Powell for the benefit of patients and the NHS.

Thank you

Yours sincerely

LH

Lesley Lyndel

Our Ref: SJP/SS-CEO NHS/15-03-21

Dear Sir Simon Stevens

RE: Action needed by NHS England for recognition and treatment of Hyperparathyroidism

I am writing to support Sallie Powell, the Founder/CEO of Hyperparathyroid UK Action4Chamge. I am one of the members to whom she refers in her letter dated 15-03-2021 and I ask you to read this letter and others being sent to you today by other members.

My GP having retired, in May 2018, I went to see Dr Taylor, a different GP in the same practice. At the first appointment, he suggested doing some blood tests. He said: "Let me see whether there's anything other than ME that I can help you with" or words to that effect. I was diagnosed with ME twenty years or so earlier, and been a patient at the Royal Free Hospital fatigue department. I am grateful for Dr Taylor's curiosity, interest, and his belief in me as a patient. A few days later, he phoned to tell say my calcium level was slightly raised (2.75mmol/L adjusted), and he wanted to repeat the test along with PTH and vitamin D.

The results were 2.64 calcium, and 8.1 PTH. He referred me immediately to endocrinology at the RFH, where I saw Professor Bouloux, in September 2018, who arranged further tests, including scans. In November he confirmed I had PHPT, and there was a large adenoma visible on the scans. He asked whether I'd like surgery. I agreed. He introduced me to Mr Law, the surgeon, who explained everything clearly and confirmed he would perform the surgery himself at the end of January 2019. Afterwards Mr Law commented that it had taken more than a few years for the adenoma to grow to the size it was; 2.5 centimetres. I had calcium levels checked in 2015 which were 2.53, 2.63 and 2.55. At the time my previous GP said they were normal, but she hadn't checked PTH. By the time I saw Prof Bouloux, I had no idea how symptomatic I was.

I had the ME/CFS diagnosis and everything was assumed to be that, until Dr Taylor reviewed my case. I have now been diagnosed with HSD/EDS, cochlear hearing loss and APD. I am receiving treatment to manage these conditions, which cause fatigue and brain fatigue/fog, as well as pain from HSD/EDS. I still have ME/CFS, either Prof Bouloux, Mr Law or both of them (I can't remember) told me clearly that even after the surgery I would still have ME/CFS.

Some symptoms cleared up overnight, e.g. I wasn't aware of how much water I drank and how often I urinated and that it wasn't normal. Prof Bouloux did ask me about symptoms when I first saw him and I just looked at him blankly. Fortunately the blood tests spoke for themselves and scans showed the adenoma clearly.

Mr Law used IOPTH monitoring and the PTH levels dropped when he removed the adenoma. It wasn't until a while after the surgery that I discovered the Hyperparathyroid UK group. Their aftercare advice has been invaluable and sadly lacking from the NHS. I have read many stories of the difficulties people in the group have had in being diagnosed, and even once diagnosed, still being told to 'wait and see'. It defies logic to delay surgery for a condition which in most cases can be cured by a parathyroidectomy, when the delay causes untold damage to the body. As well as the human cost to health, relationships and career, the financial cost to the NHS must be high, treating the steadily worsening symptoms of the disease.

Although my PHPT journey, from the time of the GP consultation with Dr Taylor to the surgery, was so good as to sound fictional, I also can't help wondering how different my life might have been had the condition been diagnosed and treated sooner. Even three years would have made an immeasurable difference to my life.

Regards

Lesley G Benedict Lyndel

Lorraine

Dear Simon Stevens

I am writing to you about my experience of hyperparathyroid disease. I have felt ill for many years and put it down to getting older, high blood pressure, gallstones, until recently in September 2020 I became very ill and very scared I actually thought I was dying.

I was having quite severe palpitations, feeling very weak, light headed, fatigued, the list goes on and on. I rang my GP and they sent me for blood tests. When the tests came back, they asked me to repeat the bloods which I did, and I got the following results; Vitamin D 35.6, Parathyroid 12.3 (1.6 - 6.9), Calcium 2.56 (2.2 -2.6).

My GP rang me, and said, 'You have hyperparathyroidism', and referred me to an endocrinologist, who contacted me on the 22nd December 2020 by telephone. He said I had mild hyperparathyroidism and mild, border line hypercalcaemia. There is no such thing as mild hyperparathyroidism. Since my diagnosis I have been so unwell. I have not heard anything since December from my endocrinologist. I suffer every day.

I have no quality of life.

I have seen my GP more in this past 6months than I have most of my life, and I am getting nowhere with anybody. This past week alone, I am in pain, and weak. I feel I have not slept for a long time.

This disease is dangerous and can be fatal. The doctors and surgeons need more training and more input on this matter, and rather than letting people suffer, it must surely be more practical to treat people and get them diagnosed quicker and safer, so it does not cost the NHS more funds, and that patients are not suffering for months, maybe years.

Update: 20th April 2021: I am so angry. I just had a face to face with endocrinologist and what a joke. I got angry with him as he is now saying my symptoms are to do with anxiety and I shouldn't take my results into account, but keep taking vitamin D. I was sobbing, and said to him, 'Are you serious? I feel shocking 24/7 most days'. He replied, 'Yes, anxiety and not enough sleep can make you feel fatigued'. I am so upset with him. I also brought up a few things I had learnt along the way, i.e. NICE guidelines, and test results fluctuating. I am seriously fed up although arguing with him, he did agree to a 24hr urine collection.

Oct 2020	April 2021
Vit D 35.6	Vit D 34.2
Cal 2.63 (2.2-2.6)	Cal 2.51
PTH 12.3 (1.6-6.9)	PTH 12.7

Kind Regards

LORRAINE

Lesley Halliday

Dear Sir Simon Stevens,

Ref: SJP/SS-CEH NHS/150321

You should have received a letter from the CEO of Hyperparathyroid UK Action4Change.

This is my parathyroid Story.

I went to my GP in November 2017 complaining of pain in my neck and shoulders. So began months of blood tests showing high blood calcium and low vitamin D, and then stopping and taking of vitamin D supplements. Each time I took vitamin D, the levels increased, and each time I stopped, the levels went down again. However, throughout all of this my calcium levels remained elevated>2.7mmol/L).

In August 2018, my parathyroid hormone level was tested and recorded at 6.2 pmol/L. My GP said this was of little concern and he would continue to monitor my calcium and vitamin D Levels.

In August 2019, I saw a different GP for repeat tests. This time the parathyroid hormone level was elevated at 8.6 pmol/L. My calcium levels continued to be elevated, the highest level being 2.9 mmol/L. My GP continued to monitor my PTH, calcium and vitamin D until December 2019, when my PTH was 9.7 pmol, calcium was 2.87 mmol/l and vitamin D was 29 nmol/L. I suggested to my GP that I might have hyperparathyroidism after researching the causes of hypercalcemia and coming across a post from Dr Norman in the US, on a site called parathyroid.com.

In February 2020, my GP referred me for an ultrasound of my neck, which showed a lesion suggestive of a parathyroid adenoma, and multinodular goitre. My GP advised I needed surgery and referred me to an endocrinologist at my local Hospital. I am symptomatic of primary hyperparathyroidism. I have pain in my joints and muscles, brain fog, poor concentration, headaches, and bouts of constipation. I also have end organ damage in the form of osteoporosis. During my telephone consultation, the endocrinologist asked if I had headaches or constipation which I confirmed. He didn't ask about any other symptoms. He referred me for a dexa bone density scan, a sestamibi scan and an ultrasound of my kidneys. The bone density scan revealed osteoporosis which he tried to pass off as due to being post-menopausal and because I went through menopause in my forties, which wasn't true. I'd told him it was my fifties.

In September I tested negatively for Familial Hypocalciuria Hypercalcemia (FHH) and was told I would be referred for surgery. NICE guidelines advise that my symptoms and blood levels indicate hyperparathyroidism and surgery is necessary. My bloods were testing again with the FHH test. The results were; calcium 2.81 mmol/L PTH 9 pmol/L, and vitamin D 46.1 nmol/L. I was sent a routine endocrinology appointment for the fourth of January 2021. The phone didn't ring. When I called to ask what happened, they said they had tried to call and gave me another appointment on the first of February 2021.

All this time since 2017, my symptoms have been getting worse, I am in pain every day, I don't sleep. My concentration is poor. I am irritable. I have headaches every day. My job and my social life have/are suffering. I have no quality of life. I am sixty one, but I feel ninety.

Following the 'missed' appointment, I wrote to the endocrinologist explaining how ill I was and that I felt he was reluctant to refer me for surgery. He phoned me out of the blue and said 'if that is what you really want, I will refer you to your chosen surgeon'. On the twenty first of January, I received a letter confirming this action. By the eighth of February, I had my first appointment with the surgeon. I am now on a waiting list for surgery.

Throughout the time dealing with the endocrinologist, he never once mentioned a diagnosis of primary hyperparathyroidism. My first letter from the surgeon reads; Lesley has primary hyperparathyroidism, which is biochemically confirmed. This was picked up a few years ago and her calcium has been at 2.8 and as high as 2.9 at one point.

'Picked up a few years ago... A FEW YEARS AGO!! Why am I still waiting for treatment?

Many people across the UK are suffering the same fate as I am. Many have been suffering much longer than I. **It's not right!**

Our GPs and endocrinologists need to be made aware that high calcium levels could indicate hyperparathyroidism, and so they need to repeat the calcium test alongside parathyroid hormone and vitamin D. Usually, elevated calcium and parathyroid hormone is a biochemical diagnosis of primary hyperparathyroidism, although there are cases where calcium appears to be normal (normocalcemic Primary hyperparathyroidism). This should not be ignored as it could be due to hyperplasic parathyroid glands as opposed to a parathyroid adenoma. These cases also need surgical intervention.

This disease can lead to cardiac problems, sudden cardiac death and stroke. It ravages your body and steals your sense of being. Our GPs and endocrinologists need re-educating on how to diagnose this serious illness. It is the hope of the Hyperparathyroid UK Action 4 Change group, of which I am a member that you, as CEO of NHS England, can bring about change, and get all potential sufferers a quick diagnosis and cure.

Watching the news recently, long Covid has had much more interest generated, in what is a fairly new illness, and long Covid clinics are being considered. What about specialised clinics for primary hyperparathyroidism?!

Thank you for taking the time to read this, and I hope you are able to bring about some much needed change.

Yours sincerely

Lesley Halliday

Lynda woodhouse

RE: REF SJP/SS-CEO NHS/15-03-21

Dear Simon

Action Needed by NHS England for Recognition and Treatment of Hyperparathyroidism

I write in support of the above referenced letter being sent to you today by Sallie Powell, Founder of Hyperparathyroid UK - Action 4 Change. Please find a copy of this letter attached, plus an article on the late Gary Shandling, who passed away at the age of 66 from a heart attack - he had hyperparathyroidism.

This disease affects men, women and young children. I will try and condense my story. I think more research needs to be done. I have had hyperparathyroidism since I was a child: my mother still says "you always needed your sleep as a little girl" .I am now 60. I remember coming home from school as a teenager and going straight to bed and sleeping for thirteen hours! One could assume this is a teenage symptom, I am not so sure. In my mid-twenties, I had a kidney stone, which I passed at home - the pain is worse than childbirth, unrelenting.

Looking back: from then on, two of my teeth became discoloured and a root canal and veneers became necessary in my twenties. When I was 34 I miscarried our daughter at 6 months. When I was 35 I miscarried our son at 5 months.

In January 2020 I went to my GP about a lump in my neck that I'd had for two years, which is probably a swollen salivary gland. She noted my blood hadn't been tested for two years, so I booked a test - it came back with very low Vitamin D. Because of that my GP asked for another test to be done and subsequently said she thought I had Primary Hyperparathyroidism and Type 2 Diabetes. She wrote to Endocrinology for advice: "I appreciate her calcium is just below the threshold you would use when deciding intervention." My calcium was 2.73, Vitamin D 23, PTH 26.4.

The NICE Guidelines state: 2.6 mmol/L for MILD HYPERPARATHYROIDISM 3.01 - 3.40 for MODERATE HYPERPARATHYROIDISM Greater than 3.40 for SEVERE HYPERPARATHYROIDISM The return advice was to put me on Vitamin D: 50,000i.u./week for six weeks, then 1,000i.u./day for six weeks, then a blood test. In June 2020, further to the Endocrinologist's advice, my GP wrote again. My calcium was 2.81, PTH 16.7 and Vitamin D wasn't taken!

I know since joining Sallie's support group that many are turned away from their GP's in the first place because they are still working on the figure of 3.00mmol/L - this is not a magic number as you can see in my case! I had a calcium level of 2.58 in 2012, which was before the NICE Guidelines were commissioned. I think my GP may have been being very tactful in the way she worded her letter. I am indebted to her for not turning me away. I was now on the NHS waiting list. I had never mentioned my symptoms to my GP as I had put them all down to menopause - I did say in our phone conversation last June that I felt like I could just lie down on the floor. She told me that if I was feeling sick or being sick to go back to her. I still hadn't heard anything in September, so I Googled Hyperparathyroidism, found Sallie's website, then joined the Support Group - I didn't post until the 29 September as I was so overwhelmed to find some many suffering with the same symptoms, and the thought that I may have had this disease all my life.

When I did post, it was Sallie who suggested to me to get my GP to refer me to Mr Khan in Oxford. My husband has private insurance via work, and kept saying 'Go privately as you're not hearing anything' I did receive a letter from Musgrove Park Hospital for a phone consult just after I had made the initial appointment with Mr Khan. The NHS is wonderful but it needs help - God forbid we lose it to privatisation. I have worked in two NHS hospitals. I panicked, having read the risks of leaving this disease to a 'wait and see' mentality. I thought' I don't want to bother my GP again', thus I contacted the insurance company to see if Mr Khan was on their list of surgeons, he was, I jumped off the edge of the pool!!

I went to the Churchill at Oxford on the 25th of November for my scans, Banbury on the 27th November for pre-op and COVID test. I was back at The New Foscote Hospital in Banbury for 0700 hrs on Monday 30th November for my surgery. **Mr Shahab Khan removed a 'rare, giant' adenoma of six cm, weighing just under nine grams, twenty times heavier than normal. He said it is the largest adenoma he had ever removed.**

You will hear about the symptoms of this disease from all the other members writing to you today, so suffice to say this disease is bloody awful, it's on a mission to destroy your body from the inside with the one cell that malfunctions, then the others follow suit and form a tumour/adenoma. Thankfully, these are usually benign, but that doesn't lessen the damage already done. There are lots of other variations/complications of this disease e.g. hyperplasia, normocalcaemic etc. I am not under the care of an endocrinologist at the moment. I don't know what state my bones, and kidneys are in at the moment. I should book a DEXA scan, but I've waited because I don't want to 'clog the system up' because of COVID, and I haven't spoken to my GP yet - I will write to her this week.

In the past two years I have had 2 lower root canal treatments and both my lower back teeth are cracked due to the calcium being taken by primary hyperparathyroidism. I will be having a conversation with my dentist about this disease. I have flown through diagnosis and treatment of this disease by the seat of my pants - nine months! There are those that 'wait' years for the same treatment, whilst existing in pain and exhaustion. **IT'S NOT RIGHT!** I really hope you will speak to Sallie Powell because without her diligence and tenacity, whilst suffering herself, and the amazing people in her support group keeping a light shining constantly, I would still be sat in the dark….again, like many others. I also hope you will take the time to speak to Shahab Khan as he is an amazing, enthusiastic and compassionate human being. 2020 was a year we'll never forget because of COVID, but for me it also was a year I am so thankful for - I have been very fortunate. .I just want my mother (85 years), my son (25 years) and my daughter (21 years) to have the blood test now, I'm still encouraging them to do so; Calcium, PTH, Vitamin D. Thank you for your service to our NHS and taking the time to read my letter.

Yours sincerely

Lynda Woodhouse (Mrs)

P.S. We're talking about the PARAthyroid glands here, not the thyroid.

Louise Coles

I write in support of letter ref SJP/SS-CEO NHS/15-03-21

Dear Simon Stevens,

RE: Action needed by NHS England for recognition and treatment of Hyperparathyroidism

I write to you from my hotel room in Oxford where I am awaiting my surgery tomorrow for removal of two adenomas of my parathyroid. In fact there may be more, but that is what has currently been picked up over the numerous ultrasounds and scans currently undertaken.

The reason I am in Oxford, 106 miles away from my home, is that my local endocrinologist decided to ignore NICE guidelines, despite locating an adenoma on an ultrasound, and monitoring my high normal to high calcium levels, along with my raised PTH levels for over two years.

This meant I had to look elsewhere for someone willing to operate, as apparently, I am not 'severe' enough for surgery as my levels aren't 'high enough' – it seems he felt it best to wait until I had, and I quote 'kidney stones or signs of osteoporosis' before I was worthy of treatment, -.a bit like shutting the stable door after the horse has bolted really.

Please note that I am a 41-year-old mother of three, however, due to this disease, my life is not that of a person of my age.

My bones are being robbed of calcium, and I am plagued with numerous symptoms, including extreme fatigue, poor concentration, memory loss, aching bones. I fear that I do not fully comprehend what symptoms I am experiencing, and will only be able to fully understand once I have had my surgery and I am healing. In 2021 this kind of treatment is quite frankly appalling, and not acceptable.

Urgent action needs to be taken as this disease is not fully understood by many GP's and hospitals. Many people are being let down and are merely existing in life due to the severity of their symptoms.

Kind regards

Louise Coles

Lynne Kirkwood

SJP/SS-CEO NHS/15-03-21

Dear Sir Simon Stevens

Re: letter from Sallie Powell, here is my NHS PHPT story

I have unknowingly been suffering from PHPT for 10 years and it is only recently after being diagnosed with kidney stones that the real reason for my illnesses has hopefully been discovered. I have now been referred to see a surgeon but obviously in view of present pressures this has not happened yet. I am of course hoping that this will eventually lead to surgery which may change my health and end this awful period in my life.

In my case it may be that all my health issues will not be resolved because too much damage has already been done. My son lives in the USA and I have a grandson aged two. It would be impossible for me to make that journey in my present state of health. I am obviously hoping that the surgery will make enough of a difference to make that visit a reality. I mention this just to highlight the personal as well as physical suffering this condition causes.

I love and fully appreciate the NHS and everything that is provided for us. I believe that not everyone in the UK realises how lucky we are but I am supporting this endeavour to get our condition highlighted as I feel money is being wasted and suffering is ensuing because we are not being signposted quickly enough. The result of this is that the numerous illnesses that result from this condition get a chance to take hold and may progress to the extent that not all issues will be resolved following surgery. Some of the investigations I have received are listed here.

2011; Surgery for wrist fracture (locking plate)
2012; MRI Sinus, Proctogram, Anorectal Physiology Manometry
2014; Sigmoidoscopy, Gastroenterology clinics
2015; Heart clinic for palpitations, 24 hr heart monitor, Echocardiogram, Cardiology clinic

2016; Colonoscopy
2018; Ultrasound abdomen, Haematuria clinic, CT scan of urinary tract, CT scan of abdomen
2019; Urology clinic, X-rays
2019/20; Lithotripsy x 3
20/21; Following tests by renal team referred to Endo. 24 hr urine, bloods, Dexa scan (still awaiting result).

Interspersed during this period are visits to A & E and GP. It was finally my beginning treatment for kidney stones and the way my heart reacted to my treatment that the renal team (who I cannot speak highly enough of) referred me to an Endocrinologist as they suspected PHPT. In one sense though this means that it was not until I had heart problems and ultimately kidney problems that the real cause of my illnesses was discovered.

I have mentioned the word suffering several times in this letter and this cannot be underestimated. I am and hopefully will always be, a cup half full type of character but this illness has brought me to the depths of despair, and it was only when I finally had a diagnosis that this feeling lifted somewhat. I still cannot do all the things I would wish and I obviously do not know yet whether or how many of my symptoms may be improved or cured by surgery as I have been ill a long time.

This group has allowed me to share concerns and we have supported one another in the long wait for diagnosis in most cases. You only find this group however once diagnosed and so for years I suffered alone blaming separate symptoms on other factors. As a collective we are amazed what sometimes very unusual symptoms we have in common. Some may not be related to PHPT but some I fear may well be and are really debilitating as well as bizarre.

I would urge you to listen to our pleas even though we live in times when the NHS is under pressure because I am sure if people who have never complained of lethargy, heart problems or pain etc. suddenly present this should be checked as there is money as well as health to be saved by swift action. I hope you will speak to the Doctors who are knowledgeable so that you can make an informed decision about what money could be saved and how difficult it is to live with a chemical imbalance brought on by PHPT.

Yours sincerely

Mrs Lynne Kirkwood

Maxine Webster

I am writing in support of letter Ref: SJP/SS-CEO NHS/15-03-21 sent by Sallie Powell.

This is with regards to the experiences I have had in getting a diagnosis and treatment for Primary Hyperparathyroidism for my aunt.

RE: Action needed by NHS England for recognition and treatment of Hyperparathyroidism

Dear Sir Simon Stevens

I am writing to you alongside many sufferers of the debilitating disease Primary Hyperparathyroidism. My aunt who is now eighty seven years old, was eventually diagnosed with PHPT last year, but only after a lengthy and protracted process. Then it was a fight to get any action for a disease that had been stealing her quality of life and suffering, I believe for years. Years prior to her diagnosis she had suffered, numerous chest infections, always making her feel so unwell for which doctors had no explanation as to why.

These infections turned into pneumonia, on top of the extreme tiredness and kidney infections plus UTI's and strange ill feelings which were hard to explain. There was never any conclusion, just lengthy spells of being immobilised. She was always complaining of pains in her hands legs, shoulders, back, and lethargy. She was always told they could find nothing wrong.

Fast forward a few years; at times very frustrated and exasperated, as whilst she was getting older she looked after herself. We continued to complain on and off, about extreme tiredness, not feeling well, and bone pain which got worse. PHPH is known as 'Moans, Bones and groans', there were plenty of them.

Finally after waiting months she saw an endocrinologist in Nov 2018 having been referred for extreme tiredness, exhaustion and the unexplained ill feelings. She felt the medical profession believed her issues were down to her age, and why she felt the way she did. This lady is someone who takes her health seriously. She does not smoke or drink and always ate well. Her under active thyroid is medicated and has been stable for many years.

Bloods were requested only for the thyroid, and as expected the results fell within the NHS tick boxes and they could not find anything wrong. When asked about optimisation or any areas he said "well what are your expectations?" She knew exactly what he meant, her age. With no conclusion she had to endure with the extreme exhaustion, tiredness, brain fog, etc.

Some months forward, again her GP sent her for more blood tests due to her being unwell. At this time she was also urgently advised twice in one week to have a blood retest and then to go to hospital as her potassium was dangerously high as "you could have a heart attack", very worrying for her, I would describe it as too high to be real.

The A&E consultant at the hospital finally confirmed that her potassium level was fine and the unduly high reading was due to bloods not analysed/tested within a couple of hours? After which, my husband asked who is right? Yet more waste of NHS time of and resources.

Another symptom of PHPT is constant peeing as your system is trying to remove the calcium that has been stripped from your bones due to the disease, in many cases depositing calcium in the kidney as it tries to filter out the calcium. In early 2019 she had another water infection, and a large amount of blood in her urine. I had never seen that amount before, and was very concerned given her age. She also had pains on the right side of her lower back. Something which the surgeon believes could have been due to calcium. Again she was put on antibiotics, and suffered much pain along with the constant trips to the bathroom.

She was then referred to see an urologist by the GP to have a cystoscopy procedure on her bladder and urethra to check there was nothing else going on, luckily it was negative.

Later that year, June 2019, another chest infection. The GP could not explain why she was so poorly and very weak. He decided this time to arrange for an ambulance to take her to a specialist older persons unit. I can only applaud their service and care, from the consultant who was compassionate and exemplary in his care and service. The visit involved many tests including bloodwork for PTH, Vitamin D, and calcium, and where she was finally diagnosed with Primary Hyperparathyroidism. After a second set of blood tests in July 2019, they specifically requested she be referred to an endocrinologist. I was still unaware myself of the disease or its impact.

In September, as she still had not heard anything, and was suffering with kidney pain and excessive peeing. I chased the GP twice, and he decided to get her to have some more blood tests. When the results arrived he wanted to see her, sat her down and said he could not find anything wrong, he believed all were OK, accept Vitamin D was on the low side and put her on Calciferol. I chased him again a few weeks later about an endocrine referral. He said he would try, but whilst he did try, he was refused by the NHS clinical referral team, so it was out of his hands. He had even spoke with a local registrar at our local hospital whom said she did not warrant an urgent/or require an appointment at the current time, as her calcium level was not that high.

I watched as she became increasing worse and lethargic, sleeping sixteen hours a day, I was very worried and upset. However I now had more information and I requested that my aunt be referred to a skilled parathyroid surgeon as I was entitled to a second opinion. Reluctantly, her GP did not think he could, but with help and advice from the surgeon he did this. I can assure you it was no easy task having to explain and argue her case with a GP who clearly does not understand how PHPT can destroy your body and that surgery is the ONLY cure.

Many in the medical profession obviously do not know enough about the disease. This has allowed the disease to perpetuate and make life a living hell for any sufferer.

Her surgeon had already confirmed the diagnosis of the disease from blood results, PTH, Calcium, Vit D and 24 hr urine. He looked to schedule an urgent operation and requested her GP to arrange a neck/ renal US scans, and finally she got the referral to him. However, her GP still believed an endocrinologist was the way forward as he was not convinced, or even believed surgery was required especially due to her age.

There are reports published around this very issue, and it is found to be very appropriate for older people to have surgery. Strangely enough this time she got an urgent referral to an endocrinologist due to her symptoms getting worse. It was a short telephone call. Whilst initially reluctant to push through an urgent nuclear scan requested by the surgeon he did, as surgery was already booked.

The neck US was negative and the renal scan showed some calcification on her right kidney which happens to be where her pains were. The nuclear scan was also negative. However, these are only used by the surgeon to target/reduce surgery time and/or check for ectopic glands as I understand it, and for an experienced parathyroid surgeon, they are not a diagnostic confirmation, which had already been confirmed biochemically.

Her surgeon is very experienced. He knew she was already suffering the effects of the disease. Surgery took place on 17th Feb with a four gland exploration. Due to Hyperplasia, three glands were removed and intra operative PTH (IOPTH) was used to confirm cure, negating the potential need for repeat surgery.

There were very clear improvements starting the following day after surgery; cognitive ability improved, she was alert and talking, not staring into the abyss and trying to think. Some pain had improved already, but the next day she could not believe how much, considering she could not even lift a cup some days with her right arm as it would lock or hurt so much.

It would definitely appear that a "Watch and Wait" attitude until her levels had reached what some GP's , endocrinologists and even surgeons believe necessary for surgery, would have been even more detrimental to her health and potentially caused more organ damage. The NICE guidelines do not go far enough for many, and I believe they failed my aunt.
Had I not had further information found through the wonderful and knowledgeable group of people in Hyperparathyroid UK Action4Change, and medical professionals I am not sure she would

still be here, or in and out of A&E. It was pitiful watching her laying on her bed.

Once again I am astounded with the unnecessary suffering of my aunt, let alone the burden and cost on NHS system for a most common endocrine disease, which it appears, a lot of GP's and endocrinologists don't know enough about what damage it can cause..

Maybe they do know of it?!

I can still hear her doctor, "Her Calcium is only a little bit high, not that much" even the hospital registrar said this.
The analogy we have come to use is, "well it's like saying you are a little bit pregnant you either are or not, so you either have the disease or you don't."

I can only reiterate a "Watch and Wait" approach should never be option as it perpetuates and exacerbates the damage this debilitating disease has on the body with a detriment to the patient. Not to mention all the costs on various departments within the NHS. It took a specialist department with the skills to stop the drain on the NHS finances. One for PHPT would not go amiss, and appears would benefit a big saving in doing so.

I am also not sure where patient experience in adult NHS services quality standard would be on a scale of 1 - 10!!

It will be interesting to hear your response to the many sufferers of this disease, many of whom have had to use the services of various NHS departments which could have been avoided, A&E, X-ray etc.

NICE Guide lines do not go far enough and need updating, potentially delaying a sufferer gaining timely referral and treatment.

A Specialist PHPT endocrinologist who understands all variants at each hospital.

Knowledge enhancements/training material regarding the disease for GP's

I look forward to hearing from you and reviewing any recommendations that will be implemented, hopefully as a result of this awareness event.

Yours sincerely

Mrs Maxine Webster

M S

Our Ref: SJP/AH-RCGP/15-03-21

15th March 2021

Dear Professor, Amanda Howe

I am writing to you in support of Sallie Powell and the patients who are being let down on their journey. Please find below my letter sent to the CEOs of NHS England and Scotland.

Our Ref: SJP/SS-CEO NHS/15-03-21

Dear Sir Simon Stevens

I am writing this letter in support of Sallie Powell and the many patients who are being treated unfairly due to misdiagnosis, poor, to non-existing knowledge, and the 'wait and see' approach.

My journey started at the beginning of 2019 when a blood test showed low Vitamin D and high PHT after several months of worsening symptoms. I asked my GP for a referral to an endocrinologist.

After two appointments three months apart, the hospital doctor admitted he did not have the knowledge to diagnose but did arrange a CT scan because of my history of headaches and migraines. The result showed a lipoma in my brain, I am awaiting the result of a recent MRI to see if there have been any changes over the last year.

After being dismissed I then asked my GP for a second opinion, again two appointments, and even though Shahab Khan (Oxford University Hospitals) had diagnosed Normocalcemic PHPT from seeing blood test results and list of symptoms, I was told by local team symptoms cannot be caused by NCPHPT as calcium within 'normal range'.

There has been an endocrine MDT meeting that decided it is not in my best interest to have an operation. Surely that is for me to decide!

Three years ago, I was hospitalised following a heart attack and at the end of October 2020 I was admitted to hospital with an inflamed gallbladder, I have had gallstones for many years, controlled by diet. Both conditions have links to Primary Hyperparathyroidism.

I am waiting for a gallbladder removal operation. Surely, with all the scans, hospital admissions, GP and hospital appointments and numerous blood tests it would have made financial sense for the GP to directly refer me to an experienced surgeon, or are they just waiting for my next heart attack or for my calcium to raise causing even more lifelong problems?

Having now been dismissed by the hospital even though I am suffering daily, my only option is to have the operation performed privately. I did ask my GP if I could be referred to Shahab Khan but as I live in Scotland that was not possible.

I would like to know why, although we have a devolved parliament, we are still part of the UK and for most of my working life I lived in England, and if an operation In Scotland is not to be considered then surely, I am entitled to treatment by an experienced surgeon of my choosing wherever he or she may be based.

This is not a letter of complaint as I believe protocols and guidelines have been followed but maybe now is a time for change as they are not fit for purpose. I hope you have taken the time to read this email and I look forward to your reply.

Kind Regards

MS

Mo

Ref.: SJP/SS-CEO NHS/15-03-21

Dear Sir Simon

My experience of Primary Hyperparathyroidism Misdiagnosis/Surgery/Continued Misdiagnosis

I realise that this will be long, but please bear with me, as I believe it is readable, gives a lot of useful information, and is in fact quite shocking. Cup of coffee, maybe? This might turn into War & Peace!

In February 2013, I had a calcium reading of 2.63mmol/L (2.2-2.6). Knowing that calcium usually falls with age and being 61 at the time, I asked my GP to check the calcium level again along with parathyroid Hormone (PTH) from the same blood draw. The results came back as Calcium 2.6mmol/L and PTH above range at 8.53pmol/L (1.6-6.9).

Knowing it is inappropriate for both calcium and PTH to be high/above range at the same blood draw, I asked my GP to refer me to my regular thyroid consultant for her view. Before doing so, however, my GP, who had recently attended a GP teach-in on Vitamin D Deficiency, decided to try and raise my Vitamin D level as it had been shown to be deficient and the GP thought the low level of Vitamin D was causing the high calcium (**Error #1:** A low Vitamin D level does not cause high calcium. In true Vitamin D deficiency calcium will usually be low, not high. A low Vitamin D level is very often found *to accompany* Primary Hyperparathyroidism (PHPT) *but is not the cause of it.*) My GP ordered in for me, Vitamin D/Cholecalciferol tablets of 50,000IU (yes, 50,000IU) one to be taken daily – yes, daily. (**Error #2:** This high a dose of supplementary Vitamin D is not prescribed to be taken daily in PHPT, as it could raise the calcium level even further.)

Worried that a daily dose of 50,000IU Vitamin D might not be advisable, I called the hospital dispensary and explained my concern. I was told under no circumstances to take the tablets with a high-range calcium accompanied by an above-range PTH level, and that the dispensary would also call my GP to inform them of the danger of taking 50,000IU daily in my case.

My thyroid consultant ignored my GP's request to see me for PHPT, telling me that any symptoms come from high calcium, and as I didn't have high calcium, I could not be having any symptoms. Confused logic. (**Error #3**: NHS Choices section on PHPT clearly states *"The severity of symptoms does not always relate to the level of calcium in your blood. For example, some people with a slightly raised calcium level may have symptoms, while others with high calcium levels may have few or no symptoms at all."*) **Error #4**: Research indicates that a raised PTH level over time can have serious cardiovascular repercussions that sometimes do not resolve even after parathyroid surgery.

After six months of continuously raised calcium levels paired with above-range PTH readings, the lead GP at my local practice did arrange for me a neck ultrasound, at which was seen a 1.8cm potential candidate for a parathyroid adenoma. I asked to be referred to an endocrinologist at my local hospital who told me that my calcium level of 2.45mmol/L (2.2-2.6) paired with a PTH level of 12.77pmol/L (1.6-6.9) from the same blood draw on a background of Vitamin D repletion was nothing to worry about (**Error #5:** These readings indicate PHPT, especially when a potential adenoma has already been seen on an ultrasound scan.)

When informed of the positive ultrasound scan result from my local hospital, the area consultant registrar arranged an ultrasound which showed the same possible parathyroid adenoma. I sought the advice of five more medical professionals who diagnosed primary hyperparathyroidism from my blood test results:

Dr O	Rheumatologist	Local hospital
Dr L	Endocrinologist	Private consult
Dr Michael Holick	Eminent Vitamin D Researcher	USA
Dr James Norman	Norman Parathyroid Centre	USA
Mr X	Endocrine Surgeon	London hospital

By this time I was having quite severe bone pain, frequent urination, extreme thirst, crushing fatigue, and marked brain fog/cognitive issues, and so had sought an experienced endocrine surgeon who accepted me onto his NHS list for parathyroid surgery. He operated in December 2014, removing 3 hyperplastic parathyroid glands, and the intra-operatively measured PTH level only fell from 26 to 8pmol/L when the third hyper functioning PTH gland had been located and removed.

Both my surgeon and I were happy with the results of surgery. My brain fog disappeared very soon afterwards and I could drive myself home on familiar roads once again without them looking totally unfamiliar. The double vision resolved, frequent thirst/urination ceased and, although left with some residual fatigue and the bone pain which has not resolved, I believe parathyroid surgery was successful for me. I have had a small kidney stone subsequently seen on ultrasound but, as I understand the matter, parathyroid hyperplasia is never totally cured but only managed, in the hope of having a gap of – in my case – hopefully some several years before my final gland becomes hyperplastic.

Post-Surgery

My London surgeon referred me back to the area hospital for my future care, although I was hardly prepared for the situation that was to cause. Neither my original thyroid consultant, nor the endocrinologist back to whom my surgeon referred me would see me after my parathyroid surgery. (**Error #6:** This left me with no post-operative monitoring.) The reason I wanted to be seen was to be able to ask someone if, in light of having had three-gland parathyroid hyperplasia with the fourth most normal looking gland left in place, I should be tested for the genetic issues that are known to be associated with primary hyperparathyroidism. This did not seem to me to be an unreasonable request as, prior to surgery, a locum GP had voiced the possibility of MEN1 based on my medical history.

I asked my GP to refer me to the Adult Genetics Department at the area hospital where I was seen by a Genetics Counsellor and a new endocrinologist. I was quite prepared to be told that testing for Men1 etc. was not necessary in my case, but what I did not expect to be told was that I had never had primary hyperparathyroidism in the first place, merely hypercellular PTH glands due to Vitamin D deficiency. (**Error #7:** Under my GP's supervision, I supplemented with 4,000 IU Vitamin D/Cholecalciferol daily as soon as the low Vitamin D had been noticed in early 2013. My level was replete by June of that year, but calcium and PTH were both still high in their respective ranges at the same blood draw, which is inappropriate.)

I informed my surgeon that the geneticist and this endocrinologist had told me that I had never had PHPT in the first place (the implication being that he had initiated unnecessary NHS surgery) and he wrote to them advising them of his diagnosis of PHPT and his removal of three hyperplastic PTH glands. When I asked them if they were taking on board my surgeon's comments, they told me they were not, and did not agree with him because he "wasn't an endocrinologist." (**Error #8:** My surgeon was one of the most eminent and experienced endocrine surgeons in the UK at that time.

In order to prove to me that I had not had PHPT (despite their own Consultant Radiologist finding an enlarged PTH gland at ultrasound, and their own Honorary Consultant Endocrinologist suggesting that I have it removed there) the geneticist called in the slides of my removed parathyroid glands from the surgery Hospital and asked her own consultant histopathologist to examine them. Her report concurred with the surgeon's histology report that the glands were hypercellular but also added that the largest of the three hyperplastic glands removed also contained a nodule of chief cells showing no parenchymal fat, the differential diagnosis of which lay between micronodular hyperplasia and a microadenoma. When I asked the Consultant Histopathologist if this finding would indicate PHPT, she first conferred with the geneticist and then replied to me that she could not say so. (**Error #9:** Several years later, I met the same endocrinologist whom I had seen along with the geneticist, at a MEN patient information day where she was conducting the question & answer session. I asked her if the presence of parathyroid micronodular hyperplasia or a parathyroid microadenoma against a background of two further hyperplastic PTH glands indicated to her a case of primary hyperparathyroidism, she said unequivocally that it did.

This endocrinologist had left the area hospital by then. I wrote to her in her new post pointing out that she had been advising the geneticist who told me (in writing, several times) that I had not had PHPT, which had discredited me as a patient, had totally confounded my medical notes, and meant that my health issues had not been followed up. She told me that she could not help now and that I needed to contact the geneticist again.

I had a long-running correspondence with this geneticist for some time. I am a professional technical translator, so no stranger to highly technical research. I gave her the benefit of my five-years of exclusive research into PHPT (!), and of having been a member of two (now folded) patient forums and of the one still running, Hyperparathyroid UK Action4Change, which was a stakeholder in the preparation of the new NICE guidelines for PHPT published on 23rd May 2019.

The geneticist's letter to me dated 18.05.15 states that each of the three parathyroid glands are "mildly hypercellular with retention of the adipose tissue component, i.e. no parathyroid hyperplasia, which by definition is enlargement of all glands with displacement of fatty tissue." (**Error#10:** the amount of fatty tissue can vary widely in these glands, and Lipoadenoma can exist.) The letter continues that in one gland is seen "one small focus of micronodular hyperplasia or a microadenoma". Microadenoma may be rare (see the article by John Lynn entitled What May Be Found at Surgery) but are a clear manifestation of PHPT, as are multiple hypercellular/hyperplastic glands. This letter continues: "Therefore, generalised multiple gland hyperplasia is not seen". (**Error #11:** Hyperplasia affects all parathyroid glands, however asymmetrically or asynchronously.) My eminent and experienced surgeon informed me that all glands were hyperplastic and the one left in situ was the "most normal-looking gland", which he left in place hopefully to give me some further years of natural calcium regulation before the last gland inevitably turned hyperactive.

This geneticist's letter of 18.05.15 then clearly states:

"The pathology together with your biochemistry therefore do not confirm primary hyperparathyroidism."

Error #12: How can this hospital be believed when they are trying to refute my diagnosis retrospectively, and my surgeon (who was there at the time!) removed three hyperplastic glands, one of which my local hospital's *own* consultant histopathologist reported as showing evidence of the growth of a microadenoma/micronodular hyperplasia (with no intracellular fat seen in that nodule) which indicates PHPT?

Eventually I was told in writing not to contact the hospital ever again for further discussion of their misdiagnosis of my PHPT. At my request, I also received a letter listing the names of the full MDT of endocrinology and genetics staff who had taken it upon themselves to determine that there was not enough evidence to state that I had definitely suffered from PHPT, when I had already had three hyper functioning PTH glands removed.

This is shocking treatment to hide the fact that their diagnostic 'excellence' clearly failed in mine and a number of other cases of which I am aware. Goodness knows how much of our precious NHS funds was spent in trying to cover up this misdiagnosis in my case – in calling in the slides of my removed glands to be re-examined by their Consultant Histopathologist, in the dictating/typing/sending of letters to me by the geneticist over several years refuting my diagnosis, and discussing my case at MDT meetings.

All this time was NHS money.

But the geneticist was only basing her opinion on that of the endocrinologist whom I saw with her in 2015 – the endocrinologist who after she had left that hospital, agreed that I had in fact had PHPT and that I should contact the geneticist again.

It is endocrinologists who need more training in parathyroid issues. If my routine thyroid doctor at the area hospital, the honorary consultant in endocrinology who was already monitoring my hashimotos thyroid issues - had known more about the parathyroids, all this time, distress and wasted NHS resources could have been avoided.

Sallie Powell, the founder of Hyperparathyroid Action4Change, campaigned for the new guidelines for PHPT which were finally published in May 2019. They do not go far enough, however, and so our group is asking you to instigate a review of these, so as to put a stop to the cruel treatment of patients with PHPT being made to wait by endocrinologists (more used to treating diabetes than anything else) until these patients have end organ damage in the form of osteoporosis or kidney stones, when timely parathyroid surgery (the only cure for parathyroid disease) could have prevented such damage – and the further use of scarce NHS resources needed to treat it.

Yours sincerely

Mo

MYD

Dear Sir Simon,

Our Ref: SJP/SS-CEO NHS/15-03-21

I am writing to you as a sufferer of Primary Hyperparathyroidism disease as part of a campaign to improve the procedure for the treatment of this condition. Although a resident of the Isle of Man which has its own Government and medical procedures it does, as you will appreciate, follow the precedents set by the UK and the Guidelines of NICE and in many instances refers patients to England for treatment as I have been.

Delays in the only available treatment for this disease have considerable detrimental effects on the well-being of patients, extend waiting lists and a have a substantial knock on effect to financial cost to health services which could be so easily be avoided as well as the added burden of state benefits.

For myself Hyperparathyroid disease has resulted in hypercalcaemia leading to osteoporosis, extreme fatigue, cataracts surgery to both eyes and laser treatment, Hypertension and an enlarged left atrium (heart). I have experienced brachycardia due to drugs used in the treatment of hypertension, a hospital admission and severe vertigo, I have suffered a fractured ankle requiring plastering twice and physiotherapy. Dental work is ongoing. Pain is an issue daily. There have over the years been many GP & Consultant appointments, multiple scans and many blood tests.

I have gone from an independent person to struggling to look after myself. My house is dirty and untidy, I have become something of a recluse, very often I don't have the energy to get washed and dressed and financially it has been difficult. There have been times when I was not sure I wanted to go on and only the thought of the mess I would leave behind kept me going.

These feelings and conditions are fairly representative of the disease. I live alone. Others cope with young children without support or have other problems and like most illnesses it is a lonely place to be. Some stories are heart breaking.

The levels of adjusted calcium guide treatment but it is painfully obvious that patients are very symptomatic with both low and high levels and, having been left to wait, end up with complications such as osteoporosis and kidney stones. Why wait until this damage is caused and patients have endured seemingly impossible hurdles.

Sensible rationale in terms of both financial costs and humane treatment of patients must surely prevail.

Yours sincerely

MYD

Nicola Lucas

Our Ref: SJP/SS-CEO NHS/15-03-21

Dear Sir Simon Stevens

Re: Letter from Sallie Powell, here is my NHS PHPT story.
I am writing to you as a member of Hyperparathyroid UK
Action4Change; I had felt unwell for years because following a virus
resulting in pneumonia & pleurisy, I was diagnosed with dilated
cardiomyopathy in 2001 with an ejection fraction of 18%, which
was stabilised to an EF of 45% with medication, and reduced hours
at work, I also have severe endometriosis, which started in 2003 with
a 5cm cyst on my right ovary and was diagnosed after two
laparoscopies in 2004, where my womb and bowel were fused
together, and a further laparoscopy in 2015.

Following a couple of synopses, I was recommended to have an
implantable loop recorder to monitor my heart long term; -1st
Reveal device October 2011- August 2013, -2nd Reveal device July
2014- March 2018.

I went to my GP in January 2016, because I had blood in my urine. I
was referred for the following tests;
- A kidney ultrasound the same week at Basildon Hospital, where the
left kidney showed some fullness of the renal pelvis, left kidney
9.4cm, cortex 1.4cm, right kidney appeared normal in outline 9.2cm,
cortex 1.5cm, and normal sized anteverted uterus,
- A cystoscopy the following week where the consultant referred me
for a CT scan, as my left kidney was enlarged & not working properly,
to check drainage from the left upper tract.
-A CT urogram two weeks later, showed a fatty 1.5cm nodule on the
adrenal gland above my right kidney and I was referred to an
endocrinologist.

Unfortunately due to long NHS wait, and no appointments available
locally, I booked the earliest endocrinology appointment at
Broomfield Hospital in Chelmsford, the end of April 2016. After
completing two lots of 24hr urine collection tests; one with acid &
one without, the consultant, said the lump on the adrenal gland

wasn't big enough for him to worry about at 1.5cm and I was discharged but didn't receive any results.

I saw a GP in December 2016, because again, I had blood in my urine, and was referred for more tests;
-Kidney ultrasound showed fullness of the left renal collecting system and a left para-pelvic cyst.
-Cystoscopy, the consultant referred me for a CT urogram scan.
-CT urogram showed a para-pelvic cyst on the left side and a nodule in the right adrenal gland with an average density of 6HU, which can represent fatty rich adenoma.
I saw a community heart failure nurse in February 2017 (ECG & blood pressure) and was sent to A&E as the ECG showed ischemia and my blood pressure was high. The Dr said my heart condition had progressed and prescribed a GCN spray but advised me not to use it due to bradycardia, and confirmed that at some point I had a heart attack. I was discharged.

From March 2017 through to September 2019, I had seemingly endless consultations with GP, cardiologist, stroke unit, neurology, TIA clinic, entresto clinic, and A&E with endless tests and scans related to my worsening cardiac disease including; blood and urine tests, ECG, angiogram, reveal device download, cardiac MRI, head MRI, Transoesophageal echocardiogram, kidney ultrasound, sleep apnoea overnight study, and CPAP trial. I also experienced repeated blood in my urine, stomach/back pain, migraines, difficulty passing urine, vision, and speech issues, and a confirmed drop in EF from 45% to 29%. I was admitted to A&E with arrhythmia 184-209bpm, and told my myocardial infarction was likely due to a clot in my heart.

I was admitted 4th-6th March 2019 for a right posterior temporal venous infarct & started on Clopidogrel tablets. A blood test in September 2019 found vitamin B12 low 117 (120-900), PTH high 12.7 (1.3-9.3) folate serum low in range 5.9 (4.5-45.3) vitamin D low 35 (50-150). On 30th September 2019, I had an ICD fitted for primary prevention & went into aFib 200+bpm so was admitted to a ward overnight for observation. In October I was prescribed vitamin B12 tablets, advised to take vitamin D & referred to an endocrinologist due to parathyroid results.

The endocrinologist at Basildon Hospital diagnosed secondary hyperparathyroidism in March 2020 and prescribed vitamin D tablets Cholecalciferol vitamin D 800IU x 2 a day (1600IU), with a 3mth follow up blood test appointment in June 2020 which was cancelled due to Covid-19. I was discharged with a suggestion to get a bit of exposure to the sun, for my vitamin D, calcium & PTH checked in twelve months and to be referred back if any subsequent abnormality found.

Adj. Cal (2.2 - 2.6 mmol/L)	Vit D 25nmol/L	PTH (1.3 - 9.3 pmol/L)
20/09/2019 - 2.23	Vit D 35 *Low*	PTH 12.7 *High*
10/12/2019 - 2.36	Vit D 49 *Low*	PTH 11.3 *High*
12/03/2019 - 2.44	Vit D 59	PTH 8.5
14/08/2020 - 2.29	Vit D 68	PTH 12.9 *High*

In August 2020 my GP telephoned after a blood test, to say I was extremely anaemic and prescribed iron tablets. I also asked to be referred to an endocrinologist, who was treating my identical twin sister, who has had similar blood results to me and has suffered swelling in her neck.

I posted my journey on "Hyperparathyroid UK Action 4 Change's Medical group and received a response from Mr. Shad Khan, Endocrine Surgeon at Oxford University Hospitals; Shahab.khan@ouh.nhs.uk saying he wanted to help me and suggested getting my GP to refer me to him. I have spoken to him and liaised via e-mail a couple of times in the last few months. He has restored my faith in the NHS. He listens, and I felt validated for the first time since this all started. My tests are out of date, so he wrote to my GP requesting more tests. I am currently shielding as clinically extremely vulnerable due to the pandemic

- Endocrinologist Oxford Hospital 9th November 2020 Telephone appt; prescribed vitamin D tablets Cholecalciferol 5000 units (x 1 a day) and to do a blood & 24 hr urine collection after a month
- Blood Test / Urine Test 26th February 2021 (awaiting results).
- GP telephone appt 9th March 2021 because the lab refused to test my 24hr urine calcium test, as I am on beta blockers.

My calcium has never been high, so my concern is that the 1.5cm 6HU nodule on the adrenal gland above my right kidney seen on tests in 2016, has never been followed up and may have contributed to my heart & kidney failure. I have had many different diagnoses over the past five years; chronic heart failure, endometriosis, secondary hyperparathyroidism, chronic kidney disease, TIA, obstructive sleep apnoea, stroke, A-fib, vitamin D deficiency, B12 deficiency, extreme anaemia and put a lot of my symptoms down to my heart condition & medication.

Although I have previously been told I do not have primary PHPT, I have many symptoms; weight gain, despite aqua aerobics four times a week, insomnia, obstructive sleep apnoea, fatigue, muscle and bone pain, blurred vision, dizziness, restless legs, tingling hands and numbness, anxiety, depression, kidney pain, breathlessness, heart palpitations, A-Fib, heartburn, tinnitus, heavy and cold legs.

It seems that information relating to secondary hyperparathyroidism, normocalcemic PHPT, and normohormonal PHPT require further study and recognition within the NHS. There are studies in America that were published over twenty years ago. Unfortunately, the reality is that NHS patients have no entitlement to surgery, unless they have high calcium levels, kidney stones, or osteoporosis, so people like myself are being discharged when they are still suffering.

My life has changed greatly as a result of this illness, after continuing to work on reduced hours for ten years after my dilated cardiomyopathy was diagnosed, I had to give up work in 2011 for health reasons and now feel unable to work due to my poor health.

Please look at the following website: Hyperparathyroiduk.com

NICE guideline; https://www.nice.org.uk/guidance/NG132

Mr Khan messaged me a couple of weeks ago stating that mine is a very odd case, as I am on so many tablets which could be affecting how my body responds, and also isn't sure my heart is strong enough, even if he found a problem. He confirmed this on 20th April 2021, which has been tough.

I'm really pleased that my twin sister Tara's finally getting sorted and is waiting for a date for her surgery, but I am obviously worried about her too, so haven't said anything, as she needs to focus on her operation & recovery.

Until recently I was shielding (CEV), so have only had local blood tests and a telephone appointment with Mr Khan. I understand, that I've got a complicated medical history, but I am obviously disappointed, as I don't know if he can help me. I am grateful to Sallie and Mr Khan that they gave me a bit of hope for a little while.

Regards

Mrs Nicola Lucas

Nicky Herring

Our Ref SJP/SS-CEO NHS/15-03-21

Dear Simon

Re: Action needed by NHS England for effective recognition and treatment of primary hyperparathyroidism

My journey with primary hyperparathyroidism began over five years ago, where I felt unwell and blood tests showed a slightly raised calcium, which was not investigated further as it was only slightly raised. My journey took me down a route of physio, being escalated to higher physio, to a rheumatologist, endocrinologist and cardiologist.

I have had MRI spine, MRI pelvis, MRI calcium scan, echocardiogram, 24-hour blood pressure, ECG, MRI abdomen, sestamibi scan, US scan, US kidney scan, DEXA scan and I'm still waiting for an urgent 24-hour ECG from February 2020.

Having initially received a good standard of care from an endocrinologist who unfortunately went off sick, I was then stuck with a very disappointing locum whose patient manner and lack of knowledge was appalling.

At this point, I had constant, severe bone pain, hypertension, palpitations (my heart felt like it was pounding out of my chest) exhaustion, severe dizziness when walking, and severe dizziness when standing for any period of time. The endocrinologist dismissed my symptoms as my calcium was 2.69, only slightly raised. He even said primary hyperparathyroidism does not affect the heart and he just wanted to monitor me. He did not attempt to refer me or feedback an alternative explanation for my illness, I was talked over and dismissed. Almost in a bid to fob me off, he said he'd get further investigations of a DEXA scan and kidney scan. Whilst awaiting my follow-up appointment, he left and I became increasingly unwell. I was so fatigued I could not process simple thoughts effectively, I had to go on long-term sick leave from work without any prospect of treatment.

Things got so bad, that even though I am only on a low salary, in pure desperation to try and get well and not lose my job, I paid to go private, having deliberately not being referred to an NHS surgeon despite me asking, and expressing my concern about my failing health.

Now had this been a one-off incident it may be considered bad luck, however having found Hyperparathyroidism Action4Change, it is glaringly obvious this is not the case and this condition is extremely poorly managed within the NHS. Disregarding my own personal suffering, I must question the costs involved in such a long-winded diagnosis, and unnecessary investigations, rather than actually treating me for an operation that cost £4000 privately. Of that cost, the surgeon was paid £650. My operation took an hour and was successful. How much money could have been saved with a prompt diagnosis and surgery? Not only for the NHS but for the education sector, as my employer, bore the cost of paying me, whilst I was absent from work as well as employing another person to cover for me.

Surgeons will always recommend surgery as the condition will always lead to an end-stage organ disease, yet endocrinologists refuse to refer till that point is reached. It truly is insane.

 I would like to support Sallie CEO of Hyperparathyroid UK Action4Change, in raising the following three issues;

 1. The scale of misdiagnosis and misinformation to patients with primary hyperparathyroidism (PHPT), by many consultants, including endocrinologists, throughout the NHS, which causes prolonged treatment delays and can cause harm. We recognise the root is poor education at many levels throughout the NHS.

2. We request an immediate update to the NICE guideline for PHPT, published 23 May 2019; https://www.nice.org.uk/guidance/NG132 to help many patients excluded by them based on calcium levels. We consider them to be a failure and that they appear to have been

engineered to steer patients away from the NHS, and towards private care with their prohibitive surgical restrictions.

3. Immense waste of NHS resources led by poor knowledge of PHPT. To quote Mr Shad Khan, Consultant Surgeon at Oxford University Hospitals; *'Studies looking at the cost effectiveness of parathyroidectomy compared to medical management show that surgery is far superior economically overall';* https://www.surgjournal.com/.../S0039-6060(16.../fulltext

Thank you for taking the time to read my letter, I hope you will acknowledge the lack of care received by patients suffering from Hyperparathyroidism and proactively take action to resolve this.

Kind regards

Nicky Herring.

P H

Dear Sir Stevens,

I write in support of letter reference SJP/SS-CEONHS/15-03-21, to share my experience of primary hyperparathyroidism and highlight the struggles that I faced in diagnosis and treatment. I hope you can find the time to read my story.

I am a 44 year old working mother of two whose life has been blighted by this condition for at least the last 6 years, probably longer. My experience sadly is not unique, but has cost the NHS far more money than it needed to due to missed opportunities to diagnose and treat, the current clinical approach of endocrinology departments and the lack of GP knowledge about this condition.

In 2015 I had a number of hospital admissions with kidney infections. The first admission was due to sepsis caused by a kidney stone and infection. Following this I suffered with recurrent UTIs and kidney infections, and following a number of scans (ultrasounds, CTs and MRIs) a large calcified cyst was identified. I also underwent a cystoscopy procedure to deal with the recurrent infections. During this time blood results indicated that my calcium was too high; 2.72 and then 2.84 during different admissions. For some reason nobody picked this up and I was not made aware. It should have been followed up. This missed opportunity has resulted in me suffering almost 6 years of medical issues during my late 30's/early 40's, whilst my children have been growing up, which were all potentially avoidable. Prior to 2015, whilst I will never know for sure, the gall stones & subsequent Cholestectomy, infertility, miscarriages and trigeminal neuralgia that I experienced in the 12 years prior to this could very well have been linked to this condition.

I find it hard to believe that a kidney stone the size of a marble only developed itself in 2015, when we know for sure that my calcium levels were too high. This had been going on for much longer. However, on the basis that we only know for sure that I had a clear indication of primary hyperparathyroidism in 2015, I can only attribute the following health issues and tests/procedures to being as a result of this the condition with confidence: 2015-2016:

1. An emergency admission to hospital due to urosepsis caused by kidney stone and subsequent infection in Sept   2015. Hospitalised for 24 hours.

2. Emergency admission due to kidney infection in November 2015. Hospitalised for 4 days.

3. Countless antibiotics for kidney and urinary infections. I was on antibiotics almost constantly from September 2015 to March 2016.

4. Several ultrasounds, 3 CTs and an MRI in November/December 2015 to work out what the 'growth' in my right kidney was and to ensure it wasn't interfering with function. During this time all I knew was that there was a 'growth' in my kidney.

5. Surgical cystoscopy procedure under general anaesthetic to bladder and urethra in 2016 to deal with recurrent UTI and kidney infections.

2015-present day;

1. 9-12 monthly urology reviews, along with scans/x-rays, to monitor the large calcified cyst in my right kidney. At my most recent appointment in February 2021, I also discovered that I now have another small stone as a result of untreated hypercalcemia. I will need ongoing long term monitoring and treatment as a result of these stones and they cause me discomfort on a daily basis. 2017-2021 1. Anxiety and depression - medicated with Sertraline during 2017/2018 plus therapy, both NHS (CBT) and private at my own cost (psychotherapy and EMDR). Between June 2017 and February 2020 I have had a total of 5 months sick leave from work due to mental health issues.

2. Countless visits to GP because of mental health issues over the last 4 years. (Since my parathyroidectomy surgery the constant 'on edge' anxious feeling that I had been living with for years seems to have subsided.)

3. Diagnosis of reflux/oesophagitis/excess acid in late 2018 and have been on Lansoprazole since then.

4. A number of visits to my GP in the last 2 years complaining of excessive palpitations/heart skipping feeling. All dismissed as anxiety/me hyper-focusing on them until they landed me in A&E at the start of this year and were the catalyst to my diagnosis.

5. 1 x 24 hour ECG prior to parathyroidectomy surgery following hospital admission with tachycardia. The result of this was that a high number of ectopic beats were noted (and this was after I had had some treatment, and at the point of monitoring they were nowhere near as bad as they had been). The Cardiologist suggested that these were as a result of my primary hyperparathyroidism, and any decision to prescribe beta blockers should be made once I had had my parathyroidectomy. These noticeable ectopic beats appear to have settled since my parathyroidectomy surgery, having experienced them regularly since 2017 up until that point.

6. Vitamin B12 deficiency diagnosed in December 2020 after blood tests due to lethargy, recurrent headaches, palpitations and brain fog (I now know were also caused by Primary Hyperparathyroidism). This is something I am still struggling with; in particular my memory.

The problems with my kidneys have been debilitating, required a lot of time off work when I was acutely ill, disrupting a qualification I was studying for at the time, and having sepsis was a very scary experience. Not to mention two months of investigations to identify the 'growth' in my kidney and its' effect, and the worry that this caused me. I experience regular pain in my right kidney on an ongoing basis.

The difficulties I have experienced with my mental health started in 2017, therefore were completely avoidable. It is not an exaggeration to say that they have affected every aspect of my life. Socially they have changed me from outgoing and brave to someone who internally struggled with just going out for dinner with a friend. Career wise the impact has been massive and has hampered my progress without a shadow of doubt. I have left 3 jobs and a degree course as a result of my poor mental health. None of these employers wanted me to go and all highly valued me, but I was unable to see the value in myself and cope with the requirements of these roles. I am lucky enough to be in employment now, and to have a decent employer, but I am currently unable to work full time and the impact of this disease means that I may now never achieve my career potential.

At the start of this year my health deteriorated rather quickly and acutely. The service I received as a result of this, in particular from the endocrinology team at my local hospital, was at best worrying, at worst quite frankly dangerous. Timeline as follows:

1st January 2021 - after a day of palpitations that would not settle, I was sent to A&E by the out of hours GP. I was admitted with tachycardia, a high number of ectopic beats and a blood test showed that my calcium level was 3.19. One of the A&E doctors mentioned hyperparathyroidism and talked about 'stones, groans, bones and moans.' I explained that I had had classic 'stones, moans and groans' over the last 5 or 6 years. The following day I was discharged with no further treatment and the consultant on AMU referred me to Endocrinology describing me as 'asymptomatic'! A somewhat surprising conclusion given that my admission he was discharging me from was for symptoms of this condition, and my background of symptomatic years preceding this.

My husband called the endocrinology team to explain that I was far from asymptomatic and the irritated response we received was, and this is a direct quote, "**what is it you want us to do about it**?" With symptomatic hypercalcaemia and an untreated calcium level of 3.19, looking at current NICE guidelines, this was not the response we expected. My blood results showed a PTH level of 39.8, over 5 times the highest normal level, a clear diagnosis of Primary Hyperparathyroidism. After discharge I felt dreadful. A visit to my GP on 7th January after 5 days of palpitations and noticeable constant ectopic beats, the worst exhaustion I have ever known and being unable to think straight, resulted in me being sent to the hospital day assessment unit with a calcium level of 3.43mmol/L.

This turned into a three day admission. You would think that at this critical point, urgent scans and a surgical referral would be the course of action taken. Instead, with no face to face specialist input, I was given a lot of IV fluid, an alendronic acid infusion and faced three days in hospital trying to reduce my calcium to an acceptable level. I was discharged still feeling dreadfully unwell and with my calcium level still at 2.93; clearly this treatment was not effective enough and further urgent action should have been taken. I also now know that this drug is unadvisable in someone with the gastric issues that I am medicated for.

Unsurprisingly by 13th January I was back at my GP surgery having further blood tests. The doctor I saw, not my usual GP, was sympathetic but reasonably dismissive. She had no understanding or knowledge of primary hyperparathyroidism. Because I was tearful, mainly because I had become so unwell that my husband had had to dress me that morning, and help me into the car to get me to the surgery, the doctor decided that I was over-anxious, but she would take bloods to put my mind at rest, and would update endocrinology to ask them to see me a bit sooner, but that essentially she felt that I was fine and this was likely to be an issue with my mental health.

The next morning I received a phone call from my actual GP who told me that my blood results showed a dangerously low phosphate level, and I needed to be readmitted to hospital for a phosphate infusion. I now know that hypophosphatemia can be a complication of receiving alendronic acid, as well as a symptom of primary hyperparathyroidism. Having asked my GP about a surgical referral to Mr Shahab Khan in Oxford (who I had spoken to, and who felt that I was a very urgent surgical case), he patronisingly explained to me that I was getting ahead of myself and I needed to trust in the endocrinologists. He did not seem to be aware that the only cure for this condition is surgery, and in fact had very little knowledge of it at all. And he wished me to have faith in a medical team who, at this point, had never laid eyes on me and whose advice had landed me back in hospital very unwell.

I am not exaggerating when I say that I honestly felt like I was dying at this time. I thought that my 14 and 11 year old sons would be left without a mother, and that nobody would help me. I was scared to close my eyes at night through genuine fear that I was not going to wake up again. I cannot even begin to describe to you how terrifying that felt.

That week, through sheer desperation, my husband had booked me a private consultation with an ENT surgeon, who also worked via the NHS at my local hospital, with experience of parathyroidectomy surgery, as we realised that this was the only way to cure this disease. As it was, the appointment was due to be the day after I was admitted for my phosphate infusion. My husband called his secretary to cancel my appointment and explain I had been re-admitted. Twenty minutes after this phone call the consultant and his registrar appeared at my bedside on the Acute Medical Unit to see me as an NHS patient, and he appeared amazed he had not been asked to see me sooner. He explained that I was acutely unwell, and the only resolution was parathyroidectomy surgery at the earliest opportunity to prevent further damage to my health. There and then he ordered an ultrasound, sestamibi scan, DEXA bone density scan, 24 hour urine test, a renal CT, all urgently and preferably whilst I was still an inpatient.

All of these tests should have been ordered by endocrinology with my first set of blood results. Half an hour later a very disinterested endocrinology registrar appeared. I overheard him tell the ward doctor I was "not that bad" and that he had "seen worse" and did not need surgery at this point. He then spent five minutes at my bedside where he told me that I did not need surgery, I could be medicated with Cinacalcet, did not ask me any questions and did not read my notes correctly. If he did, he would know that this medication was a completely inappropriate approach for me due to existing medical conditions, and the fact that I was on my third admission in 3 weeks with symptomatic, uncontrolled hypercalcemia. He made me feel that I was wasting everyone's time and his attitude towards me was, at best, dismissive. The following day I was moved to an endocrinology ward, where I never once saw anyone from the endocrinology team. A discussion about what I was doing there and that they did not want to look after me was had in front of me at handover, my mental health was discussed within full earshot of a ward full of patients at handover, and the following day I was discharged by an on call doctor who did not really seem to know what primary hyperparathyroidism was.

I was still feeling very unwell, and when I said this, the discharging doctor remarked "well, you shouldn't be" and discharged me anyway. On my discharge notes it stated that I had been taking Cinacalcet whilst an inpatient. It had never even been ordered for me from the hospital pharmacy, let alone passed my lips. I was told to come back the following day to collect the prescription as it had been delayed. When my husband called to arrange this, the endocrinology team's response was "you've been discharged now, it's nothing to do with us, see your GP."

Completely unacceptable to insist on a treatment plan, write it on my hospital notes, then in no way actually administer the plan, discharge me still unwell and wash their hands of me, even if the treatment plan was clinically inappropriate! Thank goodness for the surgeon, who booked me in for surgery the following week as an urgent case. He had also ensured I had a neck ultrasound and renal CT whilst I was an inpatient the last time prior to surgery. The renal CT showed that my calcified cyst had grown and a new kidney stone had appeared due to my untreated high calcium levels.

On 25th January 2021 I had my parathyroidectomy. In contrast to every other experience I had to this point, I cannot state enough how grateful I am for the surgeon's care, and how swiftly he appraised the situation and put the wheels in motion to deal with this. Unfortunately because it had taken so many years to reach the point of diagnosis, my surgery was not straight forward, taking over 2.5 hours instead of 30-60 minutes. On the day of the surgery my PTH was 63, nine times higher than the top end of normal range! The parathyroid gland and growth removed was stuck firmly to my oesophagus, vocal cords, larynx and soft tissue in the neck, and required delicate and careful removal. Apparently it was the largest the pathologists had ever seen at this hospital and "the clinical picture would be keeping with that of a carcinoma."

Following the surgery, because my health had suffered so badly up to this point, I was quite unwell. I was unable to be discharged as a day case due to tachycardia, fever and being unable to swallow properly, and my recovery has been a lot harder than expected. My swallowing is still not normal. Sadly, as a result of the state I was left to get to over the years before diagnosis and surgery, and the size and position the tumour had had a chance to grow to, I now have left side vocal cord paralysis and am embarking on speech therapy, at another cost to the NHS. This will also of course involve more follow up with the surgeon and possibly more surgical treatment, and this damage I have sustained may be permanent. There will be potential medical complications for me throughout my life if this is the case. It has also meant adjustments being needed at work, and limits my career progress.

All of this was almost certainly avoidable with an earlier diagnosis and treatment. As you can see, there are a number of ways I have been let down through missed opportunity, lack of knowledge of the disease, and the approach of the endocrinology team who have added absolutely nothing to my care (in fact potentially impeded it).

Firstly, the opportunity to diagnose me whilst I was an inpatient a number of times with a complication of this disease (kidney stones) in 2015 was clearly missed when high calcium was identified in my blood results. Whether this was through lack of knowledge, a slip up, or a combination I do not know. I have made a subject access request to my local hospital to investigate this further. I could have had a straight forward surgery back then and potentially avoided most, if not all, of the health problems I have experienced over the last few years, and am continuing to experience. As well as the huge personal cost to me, this could have been a massive financial saving to the NHS.

Secondly a lack of GP knowledge about this condition, which is becoming more common, and can be diagnosed with a simple blood test. If my GP had had sufficient knowledge to be able to link up my kidney 'stones', abdominal 'groans' and psychological 'moans', then it would not have taken me becoming acutely unwell and needing emergency admissions to receive a diagnosis. I believe that an improvement in GP training and better publicising of this condition could make inroads here.

Thirdly, the endocrinology input I have received added nothing to my care or treatment. Quite the opposite, it hampered it. If we had not approached the surgeon directly, quite simply I would not have had my operation and would still be seriously ill. Their lack of knowledge or understanding and unwillingness to recommend surgery, going firmly against current NICE guidelines in my case (which as they currently are, do not go far enough to help sufferers of this debilitating condition and cost the NHS hugely), and demonstrating an inability to treat this condition in even the most acute circumstances, makes me question why their input would be required at all in the treatment of this disease, particularly where diagnosis is clear cut from the outset. Endocrinology merely provide a costly barrier to cure. Even in my acute case, they provided nothing but hindrance and additional suffering for me.

My long term care is now with the surgeon, not the endocrinology team. I very much hope that you will read the experiences of me and other people with this debilitating condition and take this with the seriousness required. Aside from the human cost, it is far more financially cost effective to cure this disease at the earliest opportunity, rather than waiting for end organ damage or serious illness. It should not have taken me becoming seriously ill as a result of this condition remaining undiagnosed for so long, particularly as my clinical presentation was in keeping of that of a carcinoma, for me to receive a diagnosis. I will be forever grateful to my husband for advocating for me, and my surgeon for seeing my case for what it was. Otherwise I would still be very unwell with a growing possible carcinoma in my neck, unable to be a proper mother to my children or an effective employee, with no end in sight.

Yours sincerely

P H

Patricia Todd

Our Ref: SJP/SS-CEO NHS/15.03.21

Dear Sir Simon

My Personal Hyperparathyroid Journey to Date

I have been unwell for five or six years, but put a lot down to my age, as we are conditioned to do – things like fatigue, odd aches and pains, feeling weaker, getting forgetful.

After an episode of extreme vomiting, constipation and bruising, things came to a head in July 2019 when I woke aching from head to toe and in extreme pain. Blood tests arranged by my GP showed raised inflammation markers and high calcium. Further blood tests queried polymyalgia rheumatica (PMR) and primary hyperparathyroidism (PHPT). I was put on steroids and an urgent referral was made to the rheumatology department at my local hospital. (This was not completed correctly, resulting in the referral being rejected.)

In the meantime, further tests were organised (blood tests, ultrasound, chest x-ray etc.), but my GP denied that PHPT was the cause of the raised calcium. I found support and information from the Hyperparathyroid UK Action 4 Change Facebook group and, through them, found the NICE Guidelines. It was only when I showed my GP these guidelines, which he did not look at, that he very reluctantly referred me to the Endocrinology Department, again at my local hospital. He did not like me asking questions about my health, was very dismissive and made it very difficult for me to obtain copies of my blood test results, at one time calling me a timewaster for requesting them. I made a complaint about his behaviour.

My calcium levels ranged from 2.6 to 2.84mmol/L, and PTH up to 10pmol/L, all out of range, but the endocrinologist said there was no need to worry until calcium levels reached 3 and over. He was more concerned about the possible PMR and would not do anything further until Rheumatology had seen me. He referred me again to Rheumatology. The appointment came through for six months' time (this for an original urgent case). I decided I couldn't wait that long, so paid for a private consultation where it was agreed the appointment should have been sooner. The rheumatologist had seen the results of the DEXA scan that the endocrinologist had arranged, which showed severe osteoporosis. He scared the life out of me by saying that if I did not take medication, I would fracture and very likely die from this.

At a subsequent Endocrine appointment I was told that, as my calcium levels had not reached 3.00mmol/L, the consultant was quite happy to 'watch and wait'. He hadn't looked at the DEXA scan results, and when I told him they showed severe osteoporosis, he then agreed to refer me for surgery.

By March 2020, I was in such an anxious state, extremely worried about the damage osteoporosis was doing to my body, that I paid, once again, for both a private consultation with a surgeon specialising in PHPT, and for a private ultrasound scan, as the local hospital one (of 5 minutes duration) showed nothing. This 25-minute scan showed the adenoma and the surgeon placed me on the NHS waiting list as his private costs in London were too expensive for me. He advised it would be a few months before I would have surgery.

This worried me even more as I had the rheumatologist on the one hand telling me I could die from the osteoporosis, and the surgeon saying I could wait several months before having surgery to cure the PHPT!

Then Covid made its presence felt, and things were delayed even further.

By November 2020 I could wait no longer. Another member of the Hyperparathyroid UK Action 4 Change group recommended a surgeon in Oxford, Mr Khan, whose costs were half that of the original surgeon. I contacted him and had surgery at the end of November. Mr Khan checked all four glands, removed the rogue one and told me that I am now cured.

Immediately I woke from surgery, the brain fog disappeared and I could think clearly for the first time in months (I had previously stopped working as I could no longer concentrate). My memory has improved and I can follow TV programmes and read books again. I know which words I want to say – I'm no longer struggling for the correct word, and I don't forget what I was saying halfway through. I am no longer thirsty all the time, and don't need to keep running off to the toilet every quarter of an hour or so. My sleep has improved, and I am no longer catnapping during the day. I am stronger and have motivation and energy to do things, rather than just sitting all day. The palpitations have eased. I have gained the 9.5 kilos weight that I lost in July 2019. The anxiety I was feeling has gone. *I have myself back again*!

I don't know of any other illness where the first recommendation is to watch and wait for further illnesses to occur, such as kidney stones, heart trouble or, as in my case, osteoporosis. Surgery is the only cure for this, and it makes no sense, logically or financially, to keep patients languishing on one, *or more*, waiting lists, when they could be dealt with and cleared from waiting list figures. Diabetics are not told to wait until their sugar levels increase before treatment can begin. Patients with chest pain are not told to wait until their heart stops before treatment is given, so I don't understand why We are told to 'watch and wait' when the only cure is surgery – the sooner the better – so that we don't impact other departments and require ongoing treatment for problems brought on by this approach. Levels of calcium don't equate to symptoms suffered. There is no such thing as 'mild' hyperparathyroidism, you either have it or you don't.

Endocrinologists and GPs have a hard enough time diagnosing and treating *primary* hyperparathyroidism, let alone the other presentations of it; normocalcemic and normohormonal, although a few good surgeons are aware. The trouble is that these surgeons are too few and are getting inundated with patients, when surely, all endocrinologists and endocrinology surgeons should be up-to-speed with what is, after all, their specialty.

I do hope that you speak with Mr Shahab Khan MBBS MD FRCA FRCS, Oxford who is trying to improve the care of these patients and with Sallie, who has organised this letter-writing campaign.

Yours sincerely

Mrs P A Todd

Rachel Everett

I'm writing to add my experiences in support of Sallie Powell's letter about the recognition and treatment of hyperparathyroidism. (Ref: SJP/SS-CEO NHS/15-03-21

I've been a Parathyroid patient since July 2019 when I first went to my GP with unexplained tiredness. 19 months later I'm still waiting for surgery.

My GP was quick to spot raised calcium and PTH levels in blood tests and followed NICE guidelines to the letter.

After this the whole process has been the most frustrating and protracted experience I've experienced with any condition I've suffered before. Whilst the consultants I've seen have been consistently kind, my overwhelming feeling has been that they considered my case to be trivial and described as "mild." It seems Endocrinology Oxford still believe that calcium levels must be markedly elevated or end organ damage to have occurred before surgery should be recommended, despite current thinking.

I was first referred to Endocrinology on November 6th 2019. I knew nothing about PHPT and so did not know which questions I should ask. At this meeting no information was offered me, not even a patient leaflet or website link. The only advice I was given was to drink lots of water.

From the general NHS website I did know that the condition was progressive, so I asked to be referred to surgery straight away. I was told that:

- My calcium level was not high enough to give me symptoms
- Surgery was not nationally recommended for the over 50s (I was 54) When I looked surprised the consultant backtracked and said that as I was in Oxford I could be considered after all.

I was referred to Endocrine surgery on 26th November 2019

A DEXA scan on December 1st 2019 showed osteoporosis in my spine.

I was given an initial appointment for Mr Mihai's Endocrine surgery clinic for June 1st 2020. Endocrinology called me on the 15th May to say this was cancelled. A team meeting had picked up the fact that my blood tests (from July 2019) might suggest FHH as a cause for my raised calcium levels. Thus surgery was off and I had more bloods taken for genetic testing.

After this I heard nothing until a monitoring, telephone appointment from Endocrinology on June 5th 2020, in which I was told there was "no urgency for surgery" and I should take Vitamin D. No further bloods were taken.

By the end of the summer I'd still not had results from the genetic testing so I started to follow this up by e-mailing Endocrinology. I did not get any information until my next monitoring appointment on November 6th 2020 when I was told that I didn't have FHH and could be moved on to Endocrine Surgery as I had osteoporosis. Bloods were taken after this appointment which showed a rising PTH level. I also had a sestamibi scan on November 26th 2020.

On December 5th 2020 I had a surprise call late in the evening to say I had a large adenoma, my Vitamin D levels had dropped alarmingly and my PTH had risen to three times the normal level.

The next call was also a surprise - I can't blame The Churchill for this as none of the letters they sent me during the months of November and December actually reached me. However it was quite difficult to have a meaningful conversation with Mr Mihai, in the middle of a virtual school INSET. Finally I appeared to be on a waiting list.

I'm now in limbo waiting for an operation date and starting to feel the effects of my condition as my health deteriorates. I do understand the extra pressures that Covid has placed on the NHS during the last year. However I think you will agree that speedy intervention in a progressive but curable condition would be a sensible option. My adenoma had been developing for a considerable number of years and had already caused me serious damage by the time it was picked up by blood tests the year before last. It's now done a further 19 months of damage, yet I still have no date for surgery.

Rachel was given a date for surgery on April 21st 2021. She had a 2.5sm adenoma removed. She is hoping to catch up on sleep but has already noticed relief from bone pain and tinnitus.

Regards

Rachel Everett

Rachel Holmes

Dear Sir Simon Stevens

RE: Action needed by NHS England for recognition and treatment of Hyperparathyroidism

I am writing to you as a member of the action group Hyperparathyroid UK

I am also a sufferer of this disease

I have been diagnosed and undiagnosed twice. The second time being on the basis of one blood test which anyone who is specifically trained in PHPT would agree is unacceptable as blood tests can fluctuate especially with those who have the disease but are classed as 'Normocalcemic' but still have the classic symptoms.

I have been sent for expensive investigations unrelated to PHPT including CT scans and Bronchoscopy

This has been ongoing throughout the last 18 months. All this time I have felt extremely unwell and have had to struggle with work sometimes feeling completely exhausted.

The lack of diagnosis threatens my livelihood and wellbeing. My life is 'on hold'

I have been the subject of derision and non-belief from members of the medical profession who suggest I am anxious or depressed. All the time I have the classic symptoms of PHPT as described on the NHS website

This angers me greatly as a simple scan would clarify my condition and qualify me for surgery which I am unable to access

I would like to know why, as it stands I would need to have end organ damage or a calcium greater than 2.85 mmol before I qualify for a surgery that would financially be far more beneficial to the NHS as opposed to spending vast amounts on other investigations

Why should I spend my life feeling incredibly unwell, have my livelihood threatened and battle continually with medical professionals who are only ignorant through a lack of training/understanding of this particular disease

We are asking for an immediate update to the NICE guideline for PHPT published May 23rd 2019, to include those excluded based on calcium levels. They currently steer these people away and ultimately into private care. What happens to those such as myself who are unable to afford private health care? We suffer the consequences greatly. PHPT can reduce your lifespan by 10 years. I have a right to a life the same as all others.

Also that there is a trained PHPT endocrinologist within each NHS Trust. This I'm sure you will recognise will speed up the process regarding PHPT patients and also save the NHS so much funding!

Fully trained staff with a greater understanding is the key here – it could save so much misery and waiting for so many people who really want to be listened to, understood and to receive the correct treatment.

I hope you will take on board my comments with a good heart and a willingness to move forward and exact the changes suggested.

It's a win; win situation

Kind regards

Rachel Holmes

Rebekah Shaw

Ref: SJP/SS-CEO NHS/15-03-21

Dear Sir Simon Stevens,

Many thanks for taking the time to read this letter in support of the Hyperparathyroid UK Action4Change campaign to update the Nice Guidelines and improve medical education to both GPs and endocrinologists. It is vital that guidance and education for professionals reflects the reality of lived experience of patients with Parathyroid disease. I sincerely hope that my own medical history in relation to primary hyperparathyroidism below will give you some insight into a very typical experience.

Exactly one year ago today I began to show first symptoms of what turned out to be Covid 19, I rapidly became quite seriously unwell and didn't return to work for 10 weeks and after that only for half days ever since. I manage a busy counselling service for students' particularly medical students in major London University. My absence has a significant impact on the service at a time when demand as you'll appreciate for young peoples' mental health services is higher than ever.

Following recovery from the acute Covid infection I continued to experience symptoms of what was diagnosed, in October 2020, as Long Covid by an excellent NHS Long Covid specialist clinic. I'm sure you've come across media reports about people with long term post Covid difficulties particularly with fatigue and brain fog, muscular pain etc. The difference for me was that many of these symptoms were not entirely new, but were in fact an unmanageable deterioration of symptoms I'd had for about 8 years. Luckily for me the extensive and thorough Long Covid consultant did blood tests and then, when they showed low Vit D and high calcium followed them up by repeating them with a Parathyroid Hormone check, she then shared the results to her Endocrinology colleagues and they diagnosed Primary Hyperparathyroidism. I was referred to meet with them and am still waiting, as due to Covid they've been cancelled twice for the appointment. I am sincerely hopeful that the Endocrinology team will recommend the surgery which can simply and effectively identify and remove any enlarged glands or adenomas they find.

The troubling thing for me is that I'd had raised levels of calcium shown on previous blood tests as far back as 2012, that's 9 years. At that point the GP simply said' it's probably nothing' and no follow up was offered, had it been, and had Primary Hyperparathyroidism been diagnosed it's possible that I would never have caught Covid because the parathyroid disease could have been cured, via surgery and my Vitamin D levels corrected years ago. I also had a low Vitamin D level recorded in 2015 and again was offered no advice or follow up, another chance missed.

As I have learned more about Parathyroid disease and its common manifestations it's become increasingly clear that this was probably the underlying cause to a range of health difficulties I'd had over the last nine years including:

Repeated referrals to rheumatologists and thence for physio as a result of Back Pain, hip pain and knee pain which reduced me, aged 47 to needing to use a walking stick- the physio brought about no significant change after three courses.

Paying hundreds of pounds over the years for private osteopathy and physio for what was assumed to be a recurring bulging disc in my lumbar spine but for which my GP could offer no treatment and did not offer any imaging to determine the cause. This caused repeated absence from work.

Referral for ultrasound scans on gallbladder /pancreas following acute episodes of gallbladder/ pancreas pain.
Repeated use of OTC antacids for acid reflux
Failure to win an expected promotion at work due to decreasing capacity and time off sick for what turn out to be symptoms of hyperparathyroidism, including brain fog and fatigue.
Referral to neurologist for dementia symptoms which in the last few years which have included leaving keys in the outside of my front door for an entire working day, leaving the clothes iron on whilst away for a whole weekend, failing to recognise weekly patients in the reception areas at work, failing to recognise close colleagues and my partner of ten years when bumping into them unexpectedly and getting lost on familiar walks near my home. These are not

trivial incidents and now seem likely to be caused by hyperparathyroid brain fog.

Being unable to continue to use the potter's wheel due to back problems -which is another income stream for me and an excellent creative outlet which boosts my wellbeing.

Discussion regarding starting HRT at age 45, advised to delay by GP. Symptoms are all commensurate with Primary Hyperparathyroidism rather than perimenopause although there is obviously overlap.

I can't help but feel that it's all too easy to dismiss middle aged women with prescriptions for HRT and antidepressant / anxiolytics but as this is the group most affected by hyperparathyroid difficulties it's very concerning that symptoms of the latter can go un-investigated and or inappropriately /ineffectively treated for so long, especially given the increased risk of osteomalacia and osteoporosis.

I'd say the diagnosis was a relief, in some ways it was, but the fact that it has caused so many issues for so long, despite blood profile alerts and symptoms which could have been identified sooner were GPs and other medical staff better educated about this disease highlights the point about the lack of awareness in medical professionals. I appreciate with non-differentiating symptoms this is hard for GPs but there is more that could be done. For instance it should be fairly easy to develop a better flag system to suggest checking PTH, Vitamin D and magnesium from the same morning blood draw following a raised calcium incidental finding.

Many thanks for your time in reading this, I realise you will have read many similar letters from people in similar and much worse situations. It would be a real step forward if change could be implemented that would help prevent some of the serious health consequences of hyperparathyroidism but in many ways it's the decreasing quality of life, its impact on sufferers and their families that this disease causes, even without the money wasted by the NHS when patients have multiple unhelpful investigations and treatments for separate symptoms whilst the underlying cause fails to be detected.

Yours Faithfully,

Rebekah Shaw [Ms]

Rob Horn

Dear Sir Simon Stevens,

RE: Sallie Powell Letter, Reference: SJP/SS-CEO NHS/15-03-21

I am writing in support of the issues raised in Sallie Powell's letter dated 15th March 2021.

I was diagnosed with primary hyperparathyroidism in August 2019 after a routine blood test showed abnormally high calcium and PTH (Parathyroid Hormone) levels. Scans at Northampton General Hospital revealed an abnormality (adenoma) in one of my parathyroid glands and also osteopenia. Although my endocrinologist did mention surgery, he deferred to what I now know is NICE Guideline NG132 – 1.3.1, citing "end organ disease" as indication for surgery and recommended to "monitor the situation for now".

I did not want to end up with kidney stones and osteoporosis before being considered for a cure, so I asked my GP to refer me directly to a surgeon. He refused on the basis that I was already under the care of endocrinology at Northampton.

Having done my own research, I booked a private consultation and shared my blood results with Mr Shad Khan at Oxford Hospitals. Mr Khan wrote to my GP indicating that I had "biochemically proven hyperparathyroidism" and that surgery was the only cure. Since I don't have private health insurance my GP was persuaded to give me an NHS referral to Mr Khan and I was lucky enough to receive a successful operation three weeks ago.

Hyperparathyroidism has serious long term health implications, and I was able to be cured only because I self-advocated with the support of Hyperparathyroid UK Action4Change. I am concerned that many other people who have this disease will just follow the advice from their endocrinologist to wait and watch when they can easily be cured with an operation. Also, surely the ongoing monitoring/scans etc. is an unnecessary waste of NHS resources. I hope you will consider my case along with the letter from Sallie Powell with a view to revising the NICE Guidelines to recommend surgery as the only option for curing Hyperparathyroidism.

Yours Sincerely

Robert Horn

Dr Rosemary Sassoon

Written by her daughter Kathy Sassoon.

My 90 year old Mumma Rosemary and her evicted beastie.

Not that big really. If an average healthy gland is 40mg her adenoma weighed 179mg, so just over four times normal size. But size doesn't matter apparently as it was pumping between 17-21pmol/L (1.6-9). Calcium was 2.8. For comparison's sake my adenoma weighed 1.8g so about 50 x normal size, and my PTH was 25 (1.6-9) pre op. So, hugely much bigger but not that much difference in output. Her immediately post op tests two weeks ago came back as PTH 1.3pmol/L and Calcium 2.6mmol/L (2.15-2.6). Now two weeks later they are PTH 8mmol/L and Calcium 2.3mmol/L. So calcium does come down if it's still a bit high post op. So happy for her. Her PTH is spiking a bit as she is now re-mineralising, but she has no symptoms yet. Partly, I think because she isn't too active compared to most of us, she had great levels of magnesium and vitamin D pre op, and she eats cheese and yoghurt every day and has a milky drink at night.

I'm keeping an eye on her in case symptoms appear and she will have another blood test in two weeks. So how is she feeling? Quite amazed. She had a stroke at 68 and a fall at home four years ago which ended up as a bilateral subdural haematoma, or bleed on her brain. She had an emergency op but the whole thing left her with a leg that wouldn't respond automatically to command to lift. She had to think it first and often dragged it if she was tired. Immediately post op the leg was magically lifting by itself and she is now walking further unaided than she has for years. Most of the time she still uses her walker but this is a big difference for her. Her mind has lost its fogginess and she is chatty in the evenings still.

My sister who lives in Israel and can only ring in the evenings can have a proper conversation with her which hasn't happened for years. Mum had been tired, groggy and often cranky by the time she called. Well, we can all relate to that can't we? I think another important factor is that instead of a slippery slope to "the end" she is optimistic again and I'm sure more will keep recovering for her as time goes on. I keep telling her this is early days yet. She is talking about writing her memoirs and re editing one of her other books that is now out of print. I haven't heard her mention her will for two weeks, and she is back on her computer answering emails. They haven't seen anything like her at her care residence. So this is a biggest thank you to Sallie and everyone sharing on here, without the last four or more years on here learning, I would never have had the confidence or persistence to lead Mum through to this point, and defy her otherwise very caring, but hopeless about this, GP. I hope he is learning from this now too. When he saw her just before her op he said to her "It's nasty having your throat cut open, you know"....

I'm sharing posts I wrote in Hyperparathyroid UK Action4Change after her diagnosis, leading up to her parathyroidectomy;;

So my Mum who is 89 has been diagnosed. Her GP hasn't sent us the levels except for PTH at 21.5pmol/L (1.6. - 6.9) and the pathologist's written diagnosis of PHPT. I have asked three times for a referral for Mum to an Endo recommended by Jayne who lives in Western Australia too. Her GP visited mum yesterday to say 'he has given the referral finally because I insisted. But there's no point as it will take months to get an appointment and it won't help as nothing can be done'. **So he is content to consign a woman who was publishing books until a few months ago to the dust heap simply because of her age**. They have an appointment available for her next week. Fingers crossed. We are people whatever our age and we deserve the best health we can have.

Edit: hmmm so the delay from the GP in issuing the referral has meant mum has missed out on this month's appointments after all. The endo's receptionist has been wonderful. She asked how mum is and when I said she is deteriorating quite quickly from a couple months ago she said she will see if the Dr will open up an extra place just to see her. Now that's a receptionist! Fingers crossed now.

We went to the Endo and he was very dismissive of Mum symptoms.

He said at her age 'the only thing to worry about is her bones so he was prescribing her bisphosphonates'. I contacted my surgeon at that point who rang and spoke to mum having seen her levels. He said **"you may only have five years left but let's make them best five years we can for you"**. He ordered a 4DCT scan for mum saying **'there's no point wasting time with a sestamibi or ultrasound when this is best at finding adenomas'** He told us which scan clinic to go to and wrote the name of the radiologist he wanted to look at the scan result

Good news for my mum eighty nine years old. Clear lower right adenoma. Minimal op, surgeon says she will be under GA for about 15 minutes which was her worry more than anything as she doesn't respond well to them now. Op on 4th February. The wonder of health insurance in Covid free Western Australia. I can only wish for the same for all of you... I will discuss genetic tests post op. One step at a time

Dr Rosemary Sassoon and Kathy Sassoon

Sallie Powell

Our Ref: SJP/SS-CEO NHS/15-03-21
Copy sent to Amanda Howe President RCGP; Our Ref: SJP/AH-RCGP/15-03-21

Monday 15 March 2021

My Personal Hyperparathyroid Journey to date.

My son was born by emergency caesarean in January 1996 after a traumatic labour. I'd previously experienced three miscarriages and was told I would never give birth naturally, so I was sterilised in 1997. I'd always considered myself a constitutionally strong person, having come through several traumatic experiences since childhood. I woke up deaf one morning aged 31 which I was told would be permanent. I lost my full time job consequently and realised my life was about to change drastically. I studied for a book keeping diploma, sold my house and moved to Derby in 2000 where I signed up for full time college courses in Art & Design, ceramics and photography.

Following the breakdown of my relationship, I was diagnosed with depression and heartburn in 2000, and prescribed seroxat and ranitidine. Calcium of **2.6mmol/L** in my medical records was not picked up on, by doctors. I had a mental breakdown in 2002 following prolonged abuse from my former partner and began twelve months counselling for historical abuse. In 2003 I resumed my college courses and set up a photography business in November 2004.

I experienced crushing chest pains in March 2006 and was taken by ambulance to Royal Derby Hospital. A&E didn't pick up on my calcium level of **2.91mmol/L** and the pains subsided. I began to suffer severe knee and hand pain later in 2006, blamed by my GP on my profession as a photographer. I then began to suffer overwhelming fatigue. I had an arthroscopy on my right knee in 2007. I gave up my photography studio and took a job in retail. I began suffering blurred vision, cognitive dysfunction and severe headaches. My GP sent me to Royal Derby Hospital suspecting a bleed to the brain. I was found to have severely high BP, but again nobody picked up on my calcium level which was again **2.91mmol/L**. I was prescribed bendroflumethiazide for four years of hell, until I found out in 2011 thanks to an endocrine secretary I should never have been prescribed it with calcium of 2.91mmol/L.

2009 was a blur of GP appointments, polydipsia, polyuria, blurred vison, menorrhea, abdominal pain, fatigue, cognitive dysfunction, terrible mood swings, sudden rage, and depression/mania. My stomach grew to the size of a full tem pregnancy. My GPs asked if I could be pregnant despite having been sterilised and still having monthly menorrhea. They suggested I join a gym despite being a size 10/12. I dramatically lost 3 stone in weight in a few weeks but still my stomach was huge, solid and very painful. I finally demanded a scan which revealed 'several fibroids'.

I had a hysterectomy in March 2010. The surgeon failed to notice I had hypercalcemia and raised blood sugar. He failed to notify me that I only had a 1.7cm fibroid and Adenomyosis. I developed a hematoma at my incision site which caused me great pain when trying to walk. Four months after my surgery I still felt terrible, and changed GP practice. May 2010 after insisting I was certain I was diabetic due to polyuria and polydipsia, a GP found I had high blood sugar since 2008 and I was diagnosed with type 2 diabetes. I gave up my full time job in December 2010, because I was just too ill to function normally let alone work. I couldn't hold a mug of coffee without great pain in my hands, or actually, even a newspaper. I sold my car to stop myself driving, as my memory and brain fog were so bad, I didn't feel safe to drive.

I was so ill by 2011 I felt sure I would die in my sleep. I was in so much pain at night from my bones, I didn't really care if I wouldn't wake the next day. I asked a friend to take care of my 14 year old son if I died.

When my regular GP was on holiday in July 2011, I made an appointment with another GP about the awful pain that my own GP had dismissed as depression, and telling me I needed to get over my hysterectomy and move on. Finally, he found I had hypercalcemia. I pleaded with my regular GP to be referred to an endocrinologist having looked up hypercalcemia. She took a lot of persuading and told me I just needed to cut dairy from my diet. The endocrinologist requested scans. I was told by the surgeon that my calcium at 2.84 wasn't high enough for surgery at that point. I asked a GP to find me a hospital that would offer me surgery. I met a surgeon in Sheffield in December 2011 who did his own scan, and agreed to operate, but there was a six month waiting list. I cried on the train all the way home to Derby at that, and told my GP I was ready for the Prozac and counselling they had suggested. I pretty much slept through most of the next 6 months.

I had a 700mg adenoma removed 01/06/12. I felt pretty amazing later the same day and couldn't wait to get home. My blurred vision, tinnitus, bone and joint pain had vanished. Over the next few weeks my memory started to return, I was able to drive again. I photographed a wedding four weeks after my surgery, full of confidence and energy. I came off Prozac three weeks after my surgery. I decided to begin looking for other people with the 'rare' disease I'd had because I was amazed at how well I was. I set up a commercial and domestic cleaning business, taking on several staff.

I discovered four hundred other people with PHPT in an American support group. I set up my UK support group; Hyperparathyroid UK Action 4 Change in September 2014.

A few months after my surgery I began to notice some muscle aches and found that my calcium was increasing but still within the normal range. By August 2015, I was experiencing some severe joint pain and suspected I had another adenoma. By 2016, my joints were swollen, my head fuzzy and I knew I had another adenoma. My BP and blood sugar were both up. By December 2016 I had to give up both my cleaning business with 42 contracts, and my dressmaking business I had just started.

Over the last five years I have seen every GP at my practice, three endocrinologists and three surgeons, but only the final surgeon in Oxford would listen to me about the effects of calcium lowering medication prescribed to me in the previous four years, and believed me enough to offer me a scan on January 6th 2021. The scan revealed a small adenoma in the same position as the adenoma I had removed in June 2012. I hoped to have surgery with Shad Khan in April 2021 (My actual date for surgery is 11th May). Over twenty two years of my life has been wasted on fighting for a diagnosis of the third most common endocrine disease.

In all of those years, I've experience two and half years of what life should be like. I will be fifty four in May and what should have been the best years of my life, have been spent fighting NHS ignorance. After dedicating ten of those years to trying to raise awareness of PHPT, and seeing so much resistance from the endocrine world and doctors, to learning about PHPT, I think it's time to ask some of our 2100 members to join together and let you know the extent of needless suffering due to medical ignorance. It is time for it to stop. Please help us to ensure changes can be made quickly for the sake of many other people out there suffering, and losing years of their lives because of poor education about this very common condition.

Kind Regards

Sallie Powell
Founder of Hyperparathyroid UK Action4Change
Hyperparathyroiduk.com

Sally Ann Blakely

Dear Sir Simon

Action needed by NHS England for recognition and treatment of Hyperparathyroidism.

I am writing to you as a member of the action group Hyperparathryoid UK Action4Cchange. I was also a sufferer of this disease and believe it is responsible in part for my current condition diagnosed following my surgery to remove a benign tumour from one of my parathyroid glands in June 2019.

I join the requests for an immediate update to the NICE guideline for PHPT, published 23 May 2-19, to help many patients excluded by them based on calcium levels.

I was a previously healthy woman in my mid-fifties, working as a personal trainer and women's health coach in Harrogate, North Yorkshire. In 2018 I ran the London Marathon in the April and was fit and well. Unfortunately, within a couple of months my health began to fail. I was devoid of energy, forgetful, fatigued and started to have problems sleeping. My cognitive memory was degenerating at an alarming rate, I did not recall the faces of people I met, even clients I had seen the week before. I had to write everything down. I would work with clients and then have to sit on the sofa the rest of the time, I was so exhausted. I have always been full of energy, with eight marathons under my belt since turning 40 and at 55 felt like I was 90 Years old!

I went to my GP on several occasions; she sent me for blood tests and recognised that I wasn't well, but could not identify the problem, putting some my symptoms down to menopause, even though I was still having monthly periods. When I explained on one visit that I got into the car and could not recall how to drive, and feared I was suffering from dementia, the penny dropped for her and she sent me for bloods again. This time to check my parathyroid and calcium levels. My parathyroid levels were very elevated, but my calcium levels were closer to normal, but in the light of my symptoms she referred me to the endocrinology department at

Harrogate Hospital, North Yorkshire.

My first visit there was hopeful, I saw a sympathetic consultant who booked me in for an ultrasound. It was at the appointment with a second consultant immediately after the scan, some six weeks later, that I came across the insensitivity and ignorance of a professional who was not fully up to date with NHS guidelines. Despite the radiographer reporting to me during my scan that she had no trouble spotting the adenoma on one of my parathyroid glands, this consultant told me that I could not possibly have the symptoms I was describing because my calcium levels were within normal ranges. She reduced me to tears, (not an easy task I can assure you) by her ambivalence and indeed by her disbelief, and this despite that fact that I had a confirmed adenoma.

I stood my ground and insisted she refer me to a surgeon, and despite her insistence I could see a perfectly good surgeon in Leeds, she eventually acceded to my request to see Mr Frank Agada at York Hospital. Finally, in Mr Agada, I found someone who recognised this disease and that I had it! Following my nuclear scan he booked me in for surgery. This took place in June 2019. The change was immediate. My cognitive memory returned to normal in a matter of days. My energy levels too, and within two weeks I had begun to run again after over a year of inactivity. It felt good to be back!

I consider myself one of the lucky ones, as I fought my corner because I am the sole carer of my teenage daughter who has autism. I knew I needed to be heard. But I had to fight hard, and this should not be the case, and I know of many of my fellow sufferers who are still trying to be heard. As a result of this disease, and perhaps in part due to the delays in my diagnosis and treatment, I was diagnosed with Sjogren's syndrome about a year post surgery, an auto-immune disease I believe may have been triggered by my PHPT.

I am joining the rallying call for better recognition of this disease by GPs and Endocrinologists, in particular that the normocalcaemic ranges that many medical professionals dismiss are recognised now as still being indicative of PHPT. Too many patients are feeling dismissed, unheard or labelled hypochondriacs, when in fact they have a debilitating disease that needs to be recognised quickly, and effectively dealt with, before many more, long-ranging issues form causing even greater demands on the NHS.

Thank you for your time reading this.

I hope it helps to highlight how serious this issue is.

Yours sincerely

Sally Ann Blakey

Sally Barney

Our Ref SJP/SS-CEO NHS/15-03-21

RE: Action needed by NHS England for recognition and treatment of Hyperparathyroidism

I am writing to you as a member of the action group
Hyperparathyroid UK Action4Change.
I am also a sufferer of this disease.

It has taken me 7 months and much of my own chasing to get this diagnosis. My calcium levels appear to have been extremely raised throughout that time and I've been lucky to have already been off work as otherwise I think I would have really struggled to maintain acceptable performance levels given the amount of fatigue and pain I experience on a near daily basis.

In the light of the Covid pandemic, however, I feel myself to be extremely lucky to have managed to secure a diagnosis and now made it on to a referred list to a local surgeon. Although that "luck" is because my results have revealed the considerable damage already done to my body, and my persistence in actually getting the various tests done.

However, through my involvement with the action group, Hyperparathyroid UK, I have seen and read with horror the challenges, trials and trauma my fellow sufferers have been through – from simply having their symptoms taken seriously; to getting a diagnosis which really only requires a simple blood test; to – and then actually being offered surgery (acknowledged as the only cure) seems to have been an exhausting battle. One that they can only win, and secure their health, by becoming experts themselves who are prepared to continually push for the right tests and treatment in a timely fashion. Having to do so, when many clearly feel incredibly unwell, that their lives are effectively "on hold", is wholly unfair. It horrifies me that so many are misdiagnosed or simply dismissed – apart from the damage to their lives, what a waste of lives AND money!

Surely it would be better, both for patients and the NHS budgets, to educate and improve the understanding of this relatively common problem? To improve the speed of diagnosis and then offer surgery as quickly as possible?

We are asking for an immediate update to the NICE guideline for PHPT published May 23rd 2019 to include those excluded based on calcium levels. They currently steer these people away and ultimately into private care, assuming they can afford it. PHPT can reduce your lifespan by 10 years – it is simple to diagnose and quick to resolve.

There needs to be a trained PHPT endocrinologist within each NHS Trust to speed up the process regarding PHPT patients and also save the NHS so much funding!

Fully trained staff with a greater understanding is the key here – it could save so much misery and waiting for so many people who really want to be listened to, understood and to receive the correct treatment.

I hope you will take on board all our comments made in good faith – and show a willingness to move forward and exact the changes suggested.
It's a win-win situation.

Kind regards

Sally Barney

A copy of this letter has also been sent to Professor Amanda Howe

Sharon Lamont

Ref SJP/JC-CEO NHS/15-03-21

15.03.21

Dear John Connaghan

ACTION NEEDED THROUGHOUT THE NHS IN THE UK FOR RECOGNITION AND TREATMENT OF HYPERPARATHYROIDISM

This letter is in support of Sallie Powell who runs the website Hyperparathyroiduk.com and associated Facebook support group. Without Sallie and surgeon Shahab Khan my health would be continuing to deteriorate. I had become so unwell my family life was suffering and I had to reduce my working hours considerably.

My GP referred me in March 2020 to NHS endocrinology. I have to date not been seen. Although my calcium levels were normal/high I was advised my Parathyroid hormone levels were high due to Vitamin D deficiency. My GP advised me that it was adjusted calcium that counted and that he did not believe I had hyperparathyroidism. In fact he told me I needed a holiday! When my levels were forwarded to endocrinology they contacted the GP to say they were not concerned about my calcium levels. Not once were my debilitating symptoms considered.

Through the support of the FB group I was able to ask questions and felt I was not alone. I was also able to contact a surgeon that some other members had received and exemplary service form both on NHS and privately. I contacted Mr Khan and had a telephone consultation in the first instance. He was able to confirm a diagnosis on bloods alone and said he would help me to find a surgeon in Scotland. Due to COVID and current waiting times for NHS operations I felt unable to continue the daily struggle. Mr Khan agreed to accept me as a private patient and I subsequently travelled to Oxford for surgery. I and my husband isolated prior to travel.

My operation went well, I had a 4 gland exploration. Mr Khan removed 3 glands and reduced the size of the 4th and smallest gland. The lab report confirmed hyperplasia. My PTH dropped from 22 pre-op to 4!

I'm not the only person to have similar experiences and think that without a doubt the NICE guidelines must be updated. For reference my highest calcium in blood was 2.63mmol/L (range 2.2-2.6). My 24hr urine collection showed abnormal calcium as 10.8.

Kind regards

Sharon Lamont

Sharon Vanderzee

Dear Sir Simon

Today you will have received several notifications about hyperparathyroidism, which I hope you have found of sufficient interest to warrant their simple call to action.

I am sure you found some of them quite harrowing, and all for the sake of a simple blood test and referral to surgery.

Today is also my 69th birthday, and I feel without any exaggeration that I've been given a second chance at life.

Up until my parathyroidectomy 4 weeks ago I had become bedridden and was sleeping round the clock to try and escape my worsening constant joint, muscle and bone pain.

I had lost my ability to earn any freelance income, had to retire early from fostering, and was unable to provide full support to my 94 year old mother and baby granddaughter.

My world closed in rapidly as my health worsened, and believing I had fibromyalgia I knew life could only deteriorate as there was no cure. I had become a virtual recluse.

A chance conversation between a friend and a consultant endocrine surgeon, who pointed out the overlap of FM/HPTH symptoms, the serious implications of hypercalcemia and the fact that a simple blood test could confirm a diagnosis of hyperparathyroidism and lead to a referral for surgery seemed most fortuitous.

Luckily I had a supportive and open minded GP who was happy to arrange this on my request, and I was accepted for surgery within a few short weeks.

I felt if any of my symptoms were due to HPTH not FM I would have a net gain.

However, to my utter astonishment I have not had to take any painkillers since recovering from my operation.

Pretty much all the health issues on my adult medical records have either improved considerably or disappeared altogether.

Co-morbidities arising from the side effects of prescription drugs I no longer need have vanished.

I now wonder whether I could have avoided the need for gallbladder and fibroid surgery, private dentistry/physio/ osteopathy/ acupuncture/optometry bills, courses off antibiotics, medications for anxiety, a 4 stone weight gain and a 30 year addiction to Prozac.

It seems vets and dentists are more aware of HPTH than most GPs and endocrinologists.

I beg you to do whatever you can, as per our joint call to action. It makes so much economic sense for our beloved NHS as well as having incalculable benefit to individual sufferers.

THANK YOU for taking the time to read this.

Kindest regards

Sharon Vanderzee

Sheree Robbins

Dear Sir Simon Stevens,

RE: Action needed by NHS England for recognition and treatment of Hyperparathyroidism

I am writing to you to highlight the fact of my own personal journey and suffering with trying to get recognition and diagnosis of the disease Hyperparathyroidism.

I have been suffering with symptoms for over a decade now, the last 6 has become much more difficult. I find myself now with many of the symptoms associated with hyperparathyroidism including stage two chronic kidney disease and bone Disease. I have osteopenia in my lumbar spine and neck. This is very painful and life limiting.

Twelve years ago I was diagnosed with **fibromyalgia.** I was referred to a pain clinic for a twelve week course. Since then I have had many distressing symptoms and tests, most invasive.

- Colonoscopy for severe gut issues/ constipation
- MRI for shoulder contusions
- MRI of pelvis for endometriosis
- Cortisone injections for frozen shoulder
- Barium Swallow for acid reflux
- Virtual Colonoscopy for bowel issues
- Kidney Scan
- Ultrasound scan for Lipoma
- Gastroscopy for acid reflux sliding hernia
- Dermatology clinic for hair loss
- Physiotherapy for frozen shoulder
- Referral to A&E Eye Hospital for eye issues including vitreous posterior detachment

After feeling suicidal because of pain, I self-referred to a local government funded group for therapy. And sought help from my GP. He told me I had an adenoma on my parathyroid, Oct 2019 because of a raised blood calcium level.

However since then because my Calcium level was 2.66mmol/L and not seen as high enough by my local NHS Trust Pathology lab at Weston hospital, they would not test the three required bloods that I need to diagnose hyperparathyroid disease. I have found it almost impossible to get recognition and help from my GP surgery as they are bound by outdated legislation and budget restrictions. To date I have been unable to get the three bloods drawn together, calcium, vitamin D and parathyroid. My local NHS Trust only allows one vitamin D blood sample to be taken per year and, the lab despite the doctor requesting parathyroid would not test as it was not above 2.85, it had been 2.66.

I have had four doctors within my surgery because they either cannot or will not believe that I have this condition my health is failing. I'm in constant pain I cannot work and I am on benefits my health is declining and I will become and I'm already a drain on the NHS finances, society and my family.

I have had numerous tests scans etc. which if this disease had been recognised at the beginning much distress and financial burden would have been avoided for myself and government departments. The only support and guidance I have received is by seeking and joining an online forum and support group set up by Sallie Powell to help people like myself inform and empower ourselves.

I'd also bring to your attention the collateral damage caused by this disease on my personal life. My marriage ended after 27 years, and I'm now divorced. At 65 and without my state pension I may add, it's a huge financial burden, that's without the emotional or physical burden of being alone.

Kind regards

Sheree Robbins

<u>S H</u>

15 March 2021

Our Ref: SJP/SS-CEO NHS/15-03-21

Dear Sir Simon Stevens

RE: Action needed by NHS England for recognition and treatment of Hyperparathyroidism

I am writing in support of the above referenced letter sent to you by Sallie Powell, Founder/CEO of Hyperparathyroid UK. I enclose a copy.

I hope you will find the time to read my story, and that you can try and understand what I, and many other people have suffered because of the struggle to get a diagnosis of Hyperparathyroidism (HPTH) and then receive the surgery that will cure it.

I found out only recently that my calcium has been elevated since at least 2016. I don't have access to records before that date, but I had been in declining health for many years. At the end of 2018, I was experiencing severe acid reflux and also hair loss. My pain had become so bad, I had to sit to shower and dress. I had a gastroscopy and was diagnosed with acid reflux. I also had fatigue, a dry mouth, excessive thirst, insomnia, arrhythmia, and skin rash and hair loss.

Following a blood test, my GP said she thought I had HPTH, then after a further blood test, dismissed it. I now know that calcium can fluctuate. I believe I should have been monitored closely from this point on. I was prescribed with Vitamin D, and sometime later I was referred to an endocrinologist. I was under the impression the referral was for my exhaustion, but a later letter said it was for hair loss. I didn't know what was

In June 2019 I saw the endocrinologist, who NEVER mentioned HPTH, and was more concerned that I was a bit overweight. My husband and I were astonished that he asked me what blood tests I wanted. It was a very uncomfortable appointment. I know I was tested for Hypothyroidism at this point because it had recently been revealed to me that I had been sub clinical for a long time. He also suggested Androgens for my hair loss, even though I had a slightly elevated testosterone level. It was suggested that I have a review in a few months.

In February 2020, I had blood tests at my GP Surgery on two occasions when they failed to collect the serum parathyroid hormone (PTH) correctly and my calcium was high, so the correct diagnosis wasn't made. This was a devastating delay for me. I didn't know about this until much later as my surgery didn't tell me what they were looking at, and PHPT had previously been discounted.

I continued to feel increasingly unwell. I didn't want to live any more. I spent each night sat on the side of the bed hanging my head in despair. I couldn't talk, think, laugh, or move easily, and so on! I begged my husband of 50 years to leave me. I sold my car because I couldn't drive. I once forgot which pedals to use in a supermarket car park. I though the car had broken down and called my husband. He came to help me, but correctly guessed that it was because I was so confused. I resorted to using a mobility scooter if I really needed to go out. I stopped seeing friends. It seemed that normal life for me was over. I repeatedly told my husband that I couldn't live feeling so ill. I was in so much pain. He told me much later that he had thought how he was going to tell our son that I had taken my own life. It really was that bad! I wanted to die!

Now fast forward to June 2020, twelve months since my last appointment with the endocrinologist. I had a telephone call out of the blue from him saying he thought I had HPTH, and he wanted immediate blood tests. What had prompted him to ring me 12 months later, I don't know, but all I could think about was that maybe now I had an answer as to why I was so ill. The blood tests confirmed the diagnosis. During that year of waiting, my health had continued to deteriorate. By now, I had got to the point where I could hardly speak. It was so difficult because all I could say was that I felt ill and wanted to die. Thank goodness that my husband knew the real me, and gave me all the support that I needed.

Following my confirmed diagnosis of HPTH in early July 2020, and with no prospect of early surgery, I researched and found my own surgeon. My husband and I are pensioners and we decided to spend some of our savings to have the surgery I desperately needed. It cost us £8000! I really felt I didn't have any choice. This terrible disease was damaging my body, and I just couldn't go on. My calcium level when I went for surgery was 2.6mmol/L, but I was very symptomatic, and had been for a long time. My scans showed a "significant" adenoma. I had my surgery in August 2020. As soon as I woke up from the anaesthetic I knew I was better. My brain was much clearer, I was laughing on the phone to my husband and my son.

I spent the next few weeks recovering, but then I started experiencing low calcium and low magnesium symptoms. My GP arranged blood tests, the first of which, yet again, was incorrectly collected, so I had to go back in for more tests. I was also referred to the endocrinologist again. Incorrectly collected blood tests, together with cancelled appointments meant that it was four months until I spoke to the endocrinologist. By this time, with the help of the Hyperparathyroid UK – Action4Change group, I medicated myself and within a few weeks I felt better. This group has saved my life with their support and knowledge!

When I had my final endocrinology appointment, I asked how to monitor my bloods over the coming years. I now have to have tests done every 6 months. The endocrinologist wasn't aware that I'd had the surgery, but was very interested to know how much it cost me. I told him that I still had significant joint pain but he told me that it wasn't in his area of expertise. A few days later I was very surprised to read his discharge letter to the doctor, a copy of which he sent to me. The letter stated that I told him my aches and pains are also mostly gone and I feel a lot better in myself except for some painful joints in the hands and knees which are being investigated. In fact, while my brain fog and low mood are completely gone, I still have significant pain all over my body, including most of my joints. Not once did I tell him that my aches and pains are mostly gone.

With the knowledge I now have, it is clear that I should have been referred directly to a surgeon. The diagnosis is made from the results of the blood tests. The only thing I got from the endocrinologist was 12 months of waiting, with yet more damage being done to my body.

I do believe I had been ill for some years. My sister told me recently that about 10 years ago, I told her that I had daily pain. I also have ongoing back problems. In March 2017, I had a spinal fusion. I had scoliosis and displaced discs. The surgeon at the time told me the only proper cure would be rods the length of my spine. Considering my age and general health this clearly wasn't an option. I was 65 at the time. As I have since been diagnosed with osteopenia following my HPTH diagnosis, I believe that this may have contributed to my back problems.

Today, I am left with severe joint pain. Most other symptoms have slowly disappeared, although the brain fog and low mood disappeared on the day I had the Parathyroidectomy!

I believe that early and informed diagnosis of this terrible disease would be cost effective, not only to GPs and the NHS, but also to those people who feel they have no alternative but to pay for the surgery they so desperately need.

I ask that you consider the recommendations in the enclosed letter.

Thank you for taking the time to read my story.

Yours sincerely

S H

Sue McKinney

Dear Mr Stevens,

PRIMARY HYPERPARATHYROID DISEASE

I am writing to you; as CEO of the NHS, as I believe many are being failed by the lack of understanding of the above disease by professional medics within the NHS.

I have been a member of 'Hyperparathyroid UK Action4Change', for the past 18 months. There are over 2000 members on the Facebook page which is very well informed and has the support of some very good Parathyroid surgeons, Mr Shad Khan and Mr Paul Dent being amongst them.

Since my blood test results eighteen months ago indicated I may have primary hyperparathyroidism, I have learned a great deal from the group.

This was just as well, as unfortunately I found the knowledge of this disease by the three GPs I consulted at my practice, was very poor by their own admission. They didn't even know that calcium levels for this condition have to be taken into account alongside levels of parathyroid hormone. Apparently this is common.

From a personal point of view I have struggled with this illness. Despite my calcium level being only slightly raised above what is 'perceived' to be a normal level I have felt chronically tired, regularly dizzy with chest pains and unable to concentrate.

I am fortunate that at the moment in that I do not have the more serious and most common consequences such kidney stones and osteoporosis, although my bones have clearly already suffered as I have osteopenia as shown in a recent Dexa scan.

I waited six months for an Endo appointment (which was unfortunately further delayed three months by Covid). All this time I knew she would need to refer me for scans and ultimately to a surgeon, this could have been done by a well-informed GP. We know they can do it, so why aren't more doing it?

 I have been unable to continue with my life in the normal manner and work effectively in my chosen profession as a serving police officer. I am unable to drive any further than a few miles due to my concentration levels, I feel exhausted doing simple tasks such as shopping or walking my dog a short distance (we used to run miles together), let alone deal with complex investigations and interviews of victims and suspects.

I have basically lost my zest for life, often feeling on the verge of a break down and depression. Most of our members report a similar pattern.

I was referred to an endocrinologist, but I believe if my GP had the knowledge to diagnose this disease, organise appropriate scans and refer me direct to a surgeon I wouldn't have been left suffering as long as I have. The same must be true for hundreds of people each year.

It is a fact that many are still fighting for surgery which is the only hope of a cure and they are left suffering each day from the wide variety of conditions linked to calcium blood levels.

Endocrinologists and doctors delay surgery unnecessarily, this disease is easy to diagnose by blood tests. It's generally not complex even for a non-medic like me to understand! Sadly some medics are stuck in the past where this disease is concerned.

The education doctors receive on PHPT during training is clearly lacking and dated, it seems the illness and its effects are played down.

We repeatedly hear of our members being told such things as they only have a mild form of the disease, their slightly raised calcium level wouldn't cause their symptoms or a long term problem, or it must be the menopause, let's watch and wait and see what happens. The list goes on and none of this is acceptable.

The new NICE guidelines have been a help but still fall far short of what they should be and are still misunderstood by many GP's,

Endos and Surgeons.

This whole situation is now becoming ridiculous with many of our members requesting to be referred out of their area to travel sometimes hundreds of miles to see the most understanding and experienced surgeons who they can trust to perform their Parathyroidectomy. The same goes for the surgeons who understand **normocalcemic and normohormonal PHPT**. Both classifications of this condition numerous medics do not believe exists!

Many sufferers are having to turn to private healthcare to expedite operations as they cannot live with their symptoms. Often we hear of people taking out a bank loan to fund it out of desperation.

I would urge you to do something to sort this out, people shouldn't be told to 'watch and wait' if they have PHPT. What are they waiting for? To develop Osteoporosis, Kidney disease, Heart disease, Gall stones, Depression? We have many members suffering from these diseases and yet we are still told this is non urgent and we can be put on the back burner!

The list of conditions caused by too much calcium being in our blood and urine, rather than our bones, goes on being ignored and misunderstood, whilst all of those conditions in the long term are costing the NHS much more than what is generally one operation, and in most cases a life time cure.

I would ask you to look into this matter and try and improve the lives of many people who are suffering and waiting for surgery and of those who will do so in future years.

Yours hopefully.

Sue McKinney

Susan Williams

Our Ref: SJP/SS-CEO NHS/15-03-21

Dear Sir Simon Stevens,

RE: Immediate Action by NHS England required for recognition and treatment of Hyperparathyroidism – Combined Current NHS Practices and NICE Guidelines promote a clear breach in the Human Rights Act: Article 2; *The Right to life and to be protected from Neglect*

I am a member of the action group, Hyperparathyroid UK Action4Change, and write in support of Sallie Powell, its founder and CEO, as well as other group members and fellow sufferers of this disease who have been adversely affected by wholly inaccurate and inadequate NICE guidelines, that were supposedly developed for the diagnosis and treatment of parathyroid disease, and the accompanying significant lack of knowledge and expertise in this field exhibited by medical professionals.

I suffered with this disease and endured an agonising, undignified and prolonged battle throughout my illness, simply in order to be diagnosed and receive appropriate and timely surgical intervention (parathyroidectomy: the only curative option), a battle which apparently is not uncommon between patients and medical professionals when dealing with this disease in the UK.

The prolonged, difficult and unnecessary suffering I experienced with this disease, which put my health at needless risk, was exacerbated, most notably, due to the entire host of medical professionals I encountered and the absence of any knowledge, or a significant lack of accurate knowledge or awareness of this disease, as well as its actual, often multiple, debilitating symptoms (that manifest regardless of abnormal serum calcium height, despite this being refuted by medical professionals in the UK, but stated clearly by the majority of patients and clearly noted by countries outside of the UK) and the severity of their impact on quality of life, the lack of knowledge regarding the role and relationship between serum calcium levels and parathyroid hormone levels, as well as medical professionals prevalent and misguided use of the made-up figure of 2.85 serum calcium levels.

It is important to note that the figure of 2.85 is used as a guiding light from which the majority of medical professionals navigate to determine whether a patient meets the "criteria" for surgery or whether a patient will be believed regarding the likelihood of symptoms. It is therefore extremely unfortunate for those suffering from parathyroid disease that NICE and current NHS practice wrongly dictates that serum calcium levels above 2.85 are used as criteria for determining eligibility and urgency for parathyroidectomy (along with osteoporosis and kidney disease). This is despite NICE themselves confirming within the evidence for the current guidelines that there is "**no evidence**" whatsoever to support this particular level as a guide to indicate whether surgery is required, the urgency with which surgery should be undertaken, the number and/or severity of symptoms with which a patient may be suffering, the size or number of adenomas present or how long the disease has been allowed to progress within a patient. Unfortunately, this figure has been idly included based on its historical use rather than it having any clinical relevance whatsoever.

Only through my persistent determination, numerous letters and a multitude of emails, complaints and telephone calls, whilst suffering with multiple, severe and debilitating symptoms (which didn't however include the prerequisite osteoporosis or kidney disease however), did I eventually manage to get the surgery required.

This battle finally culminated in removal of **two parathyroid tumours (adenomas). One of which had grown "particularly large", in the words of my surgeon,** so much so, that I had to also had to undergo a simultaneous, partial thymectomy to remove one side of my thymus because the tumour had grown to such an extent.

However, prior to my surgery, and according to several GPs, endocrinologists, medical professionals within A&E, as well as my surgeon, my abnormal serum calcium levels, which tests showed had been at various levels between 2.62-2.75 (i.e. all abnormal) over the years (and therefore clearly indicative of parathyroid disease but below the make-believe figure of 2.85), alongside simultaneous, abnormal, plasma parathyroid hormone results between 8.1-12.8, had resulted in what these multiple medical professionals termed "non-specific" or "asymptomatic" symptoms.

These "asymptomatic", terrible, debilitating symptoms meant I could no longer work (after 3 decades of permanent employment), which threatened by livelihood and adversely impacted every part of my home life. These "non-specific" symptoms were specifically: simultaneous symptoms of chronic sleeplessness (recorded sleep of between 18-24 hours per week for over 2 years, or between 1 and 3 hours of intermittent, broken sleep over a 24 hour or 48 hour period), recurrent waking through the night, chronic fatigue and low energy, persistent periods of nausea and regular vomiting, anxiety and depression, frayed nerves/feeling constantly 'on edge' and 'jumpy', 'fainting' episodes and waves of extreme sickness, I was also in severe pain whilst awaiting bilateral hip replacement for bilateral hip dysplasia that could not take place prior to parathyroidectomy, high blood pressure, heartburn and gastric problems, brain fog and inability to communicate effectively, sunken eyes and ghastly, grey pallor, severe muscle aches and pains in shoulders, neck and head and feeling extremely unwell, with rarely a good day, and an inability to participate in any normal, daily activities.

These multiple, simultaneous symptoms were disregarded by health professionals and I was often treated with derision and disbelieved, and treated as though these weren't sufficient cause for concern. It is therefore important to reiterate that my supposed "low levels" of abnormal serum calcium (2.64 on the day of my op) were waved away as "not serious" or "not dangerous". As stated by my surgeon, since my calcium was only *"marginally raised (at 2.64).....it is very unlikely [my] symptoms are attributable to this"*. How uncanny therefore, that despite these laughably "low abnormal calcium" levels and supposedly non-existent symptoms, that when surgery was finally carried out there were TWO whopping, great tumours, and I not only had to undergo a parathyroidectomy but also had to have a partial thymectomy because the disease had been allowed to progress for eons and one of them had grown "particularly large".

The inaccurate knowledge of this disease, the incorrect belief that the level of abnormal calcium in any way correlates with the size or number of tumours (adenomas) and the incorrect belief that the level of abnormal calcium correlates with the number or severity of symptoms, are all proof that an adequate level of knowledge and training for medical professionals is severely absent. This, alongside the NICE guidelines, which support these misnomers and inaccuracies and which push for belief in a make-believe number conjured to ensure patients do not receive the surgical treatment they require are clear proof that patients are not receiving the level of care or treatment that the NHS purports to provide, nor do the NICE guidelines, exhibit the excellence that NICE claims to pursue, and neither guidelines nor the medical training in this area meet with the Human Rights Act (article 2) regarding individuals Right to Life and Right Not to be Neglected.

The entirety of the medical professionals from whom I sought help, were in fact either completely clueless about the disease, incorrectly assumed I had a "mild case" of hyperparathyroid disease, incorrectly assumed that abnormal serum calcium levels below 2.85 and parathyroid hormones that "weren't that high" had a bearing on disease progression, the number of symptoms, the severity of symptoms, the size and number of adenomas, and were a predictor of future health outcomes, and appeared to be in agreement that there is a preference for patients to develop further life altering and life limiting diseases (such as osteoporosis and kidney disease) before there would be a need to consider parathyroidectomy.

The sheer volume of medical professionals in various GP surgeries, endocrinology "specialists" and surgeons in various hospitals, simply from my experience reveal that they have either a complete absence of knowledge or inaccurate knowledge of this disease, all supported by NICE guidelines. This has proven at best, alarming and has likely proven catastrophic to many patients. According to the medical professionals I saw, my serum calcium results and PTH levels, which anyone with accurate knowledge of parathyroid disease, merely indicate that an adenoma or adenomas are present, made very similar, inaccurate assumptions about this disease, backed by the ubiquitous NICE guidelines. For example, according to my GP surgery these results *"weren't that high"* (Dr Lane, Fairmore Medical Practice), and *"in the mild category"* (Stephanie Driver, Operational Manager, Fairmore Medical Practice) and although this was all utter nonsense, nothing was done about them until I complained.

Likewise, Dr Ahmed Abdi El Rahman, Locum Consultant Physician, for Diabetes & Endocrinology, Royal Blackburn Hospital, had assessed my abnormal blood results (which all clearly indicated the presence of tumours) and yet stated he was *"pleased to inform [me] that the recent parathyroid uptake scan has not shown any evidence of a parathyroid adenoma (mass) which might be contributing to [my] high calcium levels. The Ultrasound you had prior to this was inconclusive…..the DEXA scan (bone density scan) also did not show any evidence of bone affection in terms of increased fragility. Your previous calcium levels were fluctuating between normal* (wrong!) *and borderline high* (there is nothing such as this term – abnormal is simply, abnormal)*, which is not serious. Your parathyroid level is also borderline high* (i.e. also abnormal). *It is not at a level that would indicate the need for surgical intervention given that your calcium is not affecting your bones or kidneys and especially as the scan did not show any evidence of detectable over-activity of your parathyroid glands. Our usual practice [when there is] no evidence of organ damage is to adopt a 6-12 monthly watchful follow-up of your bone and hormonal profile"*. All again, complete rubbish, this condition is serious, is dangerous (particularly if allowed to simply progress) and despite a negative sestamibi test, inconclusive ultrasound, and negative DEXA scan, the fact remains that I had several abnormal serum calcium and PTH test results that all confirmed parathyroid disease, which indicate to anyone with the very basic understanding of parathyroid disease, that tumours are present and require removal to prevent disease progression and that were already making me very ill.

A letter from this same endocrinologist to my GP stated *"Mrs Williams does not satisfy the criteria for referral for parathyroidectomy (in a patient with asymptomatic hypercalcaemia) given that her adjusted calcium is not more than 2.85 and her DEXA scan did not reveal osteoporosis. The only indication for surgical referral for a parathyroidectomy in this lady's case would be the fact she is less than 50 years old. Mrs Williams symptoms are quite non-specific and not sufficient to warrant surgical referral for a '? Parathyroid adenoma'"*. This is unfortunately the same claptrap I had to battle throughout the duration of my fight with this disease. The supposed wise and healthful approach stated by NICE and representatives of the NHS, is to wait until patients' symptoms worsen, placing them at risk of developing further and additional life altering and life-limiting diseases, that delays in treatment and disease progression inevitably lead to.

Even after I changed hospitals, self-diagnosed myself after taking time to read widely about parathyroid disease, made contact and joined the Hyperparathyroid UK group, who correctly confirmed my self-diagnosis, and I was finally referred to a surgeon (I had to make a formal complaint and demand this), the lack of knowledge about this disease was apparent. I waited almost another year with this illness before I was allowed surgery. My surgeon, Ms Helen Doran, Salford Hospital, incorrectly stated *"Mrs Williams' calcium level was only marginally raised at 2.64. If it is still at this level it is very unlikely her symptoms are attributable to this"*. The symptoms were attributable to the two whopping tumours in my neck, since abnormal calcium levels (i.e. 2.64) do not indicate the number of symptoms, severity of symptoms, number or size of tumours (adenomas) or determine future adverse outcomes.

It is evident from the hundreds of patients that have shared clinical and experiential information within the strict protocols of the Hyperparathyroid UK group, that insufficient clinical evidence gathering has been undertaken by the appropriate medical bodies within the UK, at any time, particularly in comparison to other countries, resulting in practices and NICE guidelines (and evidently the knowledge and learning that must take place prior to medical professionals passing the required endocrinology medical examinations) that are in stark contrast to the clinical evidence and experiences of actual patients with this disease. The NICE guidelines and NHS practices only serve to prolong suffering, promote disease progression, are incorrect in their assumptions and knowledge of this disease, and are potentially detrimental to the health of patients.

In contrast, from studies undertaken using clinical evidence from the vast pool of patients who are members of the Hyperparathyroid UK group, it has been possible for patients suffering with this disease to upload and compare blood test results, symptoms, associated diseases and follow the progress of multiple group members from initial blood tests, scans, the ensuing battle against medical professionals who do not have an adequate understanding of the disease and who often refuse to acknowledge any other opinion or information about the disease, even when proven wrong, to eventual surgical intervention. This has enabled group members to more fully understand this disease and its implications.

In light of this, the Hyperparathyroid UK group provided NICE with the appropriate knowledge and information during consultation for the development of the guidelines. However, the committee unfathomably didn't use the information from the large pool of people with the disease and instead chose to use inaccurate, fairly vague, information, based on limited and poor and ridiculously out-of-date assumptions as "evidence" to back their assertions, resulting in guidelines which only serve to promote the prolonged sickness and deterioration of patients or steer patients onto the expensive path of private care.

As laid down in the Human Rights Act, the NHS Constitution refers to and strongly echoes the Absolute Rights of individuals (article 2 - the Right to Life & to be Protected from Neglect), and states that the NHS service is *"designed to improve, **prevent**, diagnose and **treat** both physical and mental problems.........it is available to all irrespective of gender [and] age.......at the same time it has a wider social duty to promote equality through the services it provides and to pay particular attention to groups or sections of society where improvements in health and life expectancy are not keeping pace with the rest of the population".* In terms of parathyroid disease this statement is yet to materialise and practices are employed that are in direct opposition to this statement and the Human Rights Act. Likewise, the NICE Charter states that the guidance and quality standards it is supposed to provide are *"based on the best available evidence and set out the best ways to prevent, diagnose and treat disease and ill-health, promote healthy living and care for vulnerable people".* NICE is *"at the heart of the health and social care system"....[it is] "responsible for providing **evidence-based** guidance on health and social care"...."to help health, public health and social care professionals **deliver the best possible care within the resources available".* In terms of the NICE guidelines for parathyroid disease, again this statement is untrue. It is extremely disconcerting that NICE, and in direct contrast to their ethos, have produced guidelines that are extremely limited, dated, selective and ignore a whole body of patient data as well as the significant up-to-date information that is available, if effort had been made to obtain it.

Therefore, in order to develop useful, robust guidelines that put patients' lives and health and well-being at the forefront of healthcare, and with reference to the Human Rights Act (article 2 : the right to life.....and the right to be protected from neglect), it can be argued that decades-old information, that is of questionable value and relies on limited (if any) clinical evidence, has no place in the development, distribution and utilisation of guidelines, particularly since it is apparent that these guidelines do not fit with the majority of patients' experience of parathyroid disease, nor contain any up-to-date information and lack any relevant patient data studies.

It is also evident that whilst these guidelines were in development, and despite the Hyperparathyroid UK Action4Change Group consisting of over 1,000 members either living with the disease or post-surgery, no one from the Committee took the opportunity or thought it pertinent to seek information from the very patients whom this disease is currently affecting or has affected. The Human Rights Act (article 2) states that *"public authorities should also consider your right to life when making decisions that might put you in danger or that affect your life expectancy"*. Danger (in this case, the unpredictable risks and threat of disease progression in patients with untreated parathyroid disease) and the associated reduction in life expectancy of untreated patients, do not appear to be at the forefront of the evidence search and subsequent collation. Hence, it is argued that the subsequent guidelines that have been produced have omitted to consider the Human Rights of patients with parathyroid disease.

From the Committee's observations stated within the guidelines, "the committee agreed that hyperparathyroid is an under-recognised condition among both the general population and healthcare professionals", yet their guidelines only strengthen this under-recognition and advocate that this remains the case. They emphasised "the importance of accurate, balanced and up-to-date information so that people with the condition can understand it and make informed choices, particularly with regard to surgery" and have then produced the opposite.

The vast majority of Hyperparathyroid UK group members have noted the chasm in terms of the lack of knowledge and expertise of

GPs, Endocrinologists and Surgeons, which unfortunately varies significantly and patients have had no alternative to seek information for themselves due to these significant gaps. It is important for these guidelines therefore to include information to raise the awareness of healthcare professionals of such things as how the parathyroid glands work, the whole raft of symptoms malfunctioning glands can potentially create (not just the few vagaries mentioned in the current guidelines) but the multiple, often simultaneous, debilitating symptoms and illnesses that severely impact the quality of life for many patients with this disease. It is important that the NICE guidelines over-emphasise that calcium levels do not rise as the disease progresses, nor are symptoms fewer for those patients with lower abnormal levels of serum calcium, as many medical professionals currently believe. Healthcare professionals must be made aware of the significant reduction in life expectancy and significantly increased risk to higher incidences of malignancy and cardiovascular disease in untreated parathyroid disease. This would not only allow healthcare professionals to be better informed to diagnose and treat patients with this disease (and show greater compassion than is sometimes currently shown) but would allow them to be better placed to provide correct information in terms of 'patient information'.

Currently, members report a high incidence of incorrect information being given to patients at all points in the system. The guidelines should have been used as an opportunity to raise awareness, since without this information many healthcare professionals will continue to use guesswork and provide incorrect information as regards this disease. Unfortunately, the committee's emphasis on the importance of "accurate, balanced, and up-to-date information" ends there, since much of the evidence gathered is extremely limited, of low value and therefore is not "based on the best available evidence" and consequently has not produced "the best ways to prevent, diagnose and treat disease and ill-health, promote healthy living and care for vulnerable people". Nor does it provide up-to-date "evidence-based guidance on health and social care....to help health, public health and social care professionals deliver the best possible care within the resources available". It should be reiterated that much of the low value evidence used, the lack of seeking pertinent information from a wide range of up-to-date sources or information from patients affected by this disease currently (Hyperparathyroid UK members for example) is at odds with the Human Right (article 2) to "consider your right to life when making decisions that might put you in danger or that affect your life expectancy".

Please note, the 4th International Workshop on 'Asymptomatic' PHPT published a report in 2014 to assert that there is "a growing consensus that surgery will eventually be appropriate in the vast majority of patients with asymptomatic disease because it is the only definitive therapy". Indeed, according to Leiffson et al, *"large population-based studies show that patients with PHPT appear to be at risk for premature death. Most of these deaths were due to cardiovascular disease or cancer. This data included both symptomatic and asymptomatic patients"* (Current Thinking on Parathyroidism, Arrangoiz R, Cordera F et al).

This same paper reports that *"in a study of 33,346 patients over an 11-year period...a 20- 58% higher mortality [was noted], often of cardiovascular disease in patients with PHPT compared to patients with normal serum calcium levels. Patients who have early surgery for parathyroid surgery have improved survival when compared to patients with untreated PHPT. Patients with PHPT have a higher incidence of cardiovascular disease (2.5-3.0 times that of the general population) such as hypertension, left ventricular hypertrophy, heart failure, arrhythmias, stroke and myocardial infarction compared to patients with normal serum calcium levels. Some studies have also shown that the cardiovascular risk returns to normal after a successful surgery, which is important for preventing cardiovascular disease in patients with PHPT. Patients with PHPT have a higher incidence of developing certain malignancies compared to the general population (approximately 2 times higher). The malignancies most commonly associated with PHPT are breast cancer, renal cancer, colorectal cancer, endocrine tumours (adrenals, thymus, pituitary and pancreas), squamous cell carcinoma and prostate cancer"* (Arrangoiz R, Cordera F et al).

I don't see how the NICE guidelines or current NHS practice can therefore be utilising resources effectively or ensuring patient care is optimised when the likelihood of requiring significantly more NHS resources and departments the longer the disease is allowed to progress and remain untreated puts patient health at significant risk of additional co-morbidities.

Similarly, studies conducted by Norman et al confirm *"patients with hyperparathyroidism have a higher rate of: stroke, heart failure, heart attack, atrial fibrillation, cardiomyopathy, renal failure, depression, shingles, kidney stones, osteoporosis, serious bone fractures, bone pain, need for hip replacement, GERD, high blood pressure, memory loss, chronic fatigue, MGUS, anaemia...cancers of the breast, colon, kidney and prostate, and early death"* (Norman et al Parathyroid.com). In addition, Norman et al also points out that *"all patients with hyperparathyroid disease will develop osteoporosis if the parathyroid tumour is not removed.... [And] postmenopausal women with parathyroid disease will generally develop osteoporosis 2-5 times faster than their peers"*.

Thorsen et al conducted a study in Sweden on post-menopausal women with hyperparathyroidism before and one year after parathyroidectomy that *"found a significant increase in bone density in the hip and lower back one year later"*.

Norman et al confirm that *"parathyroidectomy doesn't just stop the rapid loss of bone density, it allows the body to begin healing itself"*. The above information opposes the committee's assertion that "based on their expertise, the committee agreed that there was no evidence to suggest that surgery modifies cardiovascular disease risk or fracture risk". However, if surgery is undertaken early to prevent disease progression and the development of osteoporosis (as well as the various other diseases due to excessive amounts of calcium in the blood), then fracture risk is reduced since patients either won't have developed osteoporosis or it will prevent the disease from worsening and begin a reversal of the bone loss ie "it allows the body to begin healing itself".

Similarly, with regards to the NICE committee's assertions regarding renal function, the NICE committee noted *"that PHPT is associated with a decline in renal function but there is no evidence that parathyroidectomy leads to an improvement"*. Yet, makes that contradictory statement in opposition of this, stating, *"The committee, from their clinical experience, discussed that kidney stones are one of the end organ effects of PHPT and the risk of developing stones decreases after surgery"*. So, which is it?

In opposition of the NICE committee's contradictory statements a report from the 4th International Workshop on Asymptomatic PHPT stated *"after successful parathyroid surgery, bone density improves, fracture incidence is reduced (cohort studies), kidney stones are reduced in frequency among those with a history of renal stones [and] there may well be improvements in some neurocognitive elements"*.

Most significant from this information is that patients who have early surgery for parathyroid surgery have improved survival when compared to patients with untreated PHPT. These figures are significant and impactful and are unfortunately at odds with the "evidence" utilised by the NICE committee for their guidelines. It is evident from all the above that the guidelines and the evidence on which they are based is at best flawed, limited, dated, and far from excellent and at worst, potentially extremely dangerous and life-threatening to patients with parathyroid disease. It could be argued there is an evident lack of substantial, patient-related, informative data to inform these guidelines and a gaping chasm of excluded information. This could be considered a breach of Human Rights (article 2) in terms of patients' right to life and their right to life in terms of public authorities not considering evidence that potentially puts them in danger that could potentially affect their life expectancy. Surgical intervention is the ONLY curative option, this should be borne in mind throughout analysis and decision-making processes, regardless of symptoms and height of serum calcium levels. In addition, the Human Rights Act, the NHS Constitution, NHS training for medical professionals (particularly GPs, endocrinologists and surgeons) and NICE's own Charter should lay the foundation for seeking accurate, up-to-date, relevant evidence and information, that puts the health and well-being of patients first, rather than an afterthought.

It should be noted that in an assessment of over 10,000 patients with proven PHPT it was found that 85.6% had serum calcium concentrations below 2.875mmol/L and 69% of patients had never had serum calcium concentration above 2.85mmol/L. In addition, 74% of patients in the same study had at least one serum calcium concentration within the normal reference range, "again making the point of the variability seen in patients with PHPT" ("Current Thinking on Parathyroidism", Arrangoiz R, Cordera F (2016)).

I therefore reiterate that serum calcium levels are unpredictable, they do not rise as a patient's condition worsens (as the make-believe figure of >2.85mmol/L suggests and which medical professionals espouse), they go up and down unpredictably due to parathyroid disease, which makes one or more parathyroid glands malfunction. Similarly, Norman et al published a report in January 2017 following the largest study of parathyroid patients to date (20,081 consecutive adults). They assessed *"the symptoms and complications ([kidney] stones, osteoporosis, etc.) in patients that have a very high calcium and compared them to parathyroid patients with only very mild elevations of calcium....The result: NO DIFFERENCE! People with calcium levels of 12.5 (3.125mmol/L) do not have more symptoms, or [kidney] stones, or osteoporosis, or fatigue (or anything) than people with calcium of 10.5 (2.625mmol/L)"....It is the duration of calcium levels above 10.0 (2.6mmol/L) in adults over 30 that are associated with complications of hyperparathyroidism"*. This information coupled with the committee's own assertion that there is no evidence to support the dreamt up >2.85mmol/L criteria, not only eradicates the myth that patients/medical professionals need to wait to see if calcium levels will ever reach the invented >2.85mmol/L criteria, it also asserts that patients needn't wait to develop kidney disease or osteoporosis in order to be deemed eligible for surgery.

From all the above information, my personal battle with this disease and against the incorrect assertions made by all medical professionals (backed by NICE guidelines), there is a strong suggestion there is a potentially large cohort of PHPT patients who have been already failed in terms of their healthcare and the prevention of disease progression due to incorrect criteria and guidelines, and consequently deemed ineligible for surgery (the only definitive cure). This is an opportunity to right that wrong. Has the Human Rights Act (article 2 – the right to life) never been considered by healthcare professionals or committees in the development of guidelines and practice? It appears not unfortunately.

The criteria in the NICE guidelines should therefore stipulate that ALL patients, without exception and without having to reach some "plucked from the air" calcium level should all be referred for surgery. At that point, consideration can be made as to whether a patient is suitable for surgery only in terms of the likelihood of their being medically fit to undergo surgery. In addition, it would be sensible for those patients with osteoporosis and/or kidney disease or any of the other major life-changing/threatening symptoms to be given priority over those without these major diseases. However, a strict adherence to an 18-week wait from diagnosis to surgery should be maintained in order to prevent disease progression and patient suffering.

In addition, in terms of being assessed for surgery, should one serum calcium level drop, or should a patient's serum calcium levels never reach a certain height, they should not be subsequently bumped lower down the waiting list for surgery. As per the above, over two thirds of patients' serum calcium will never reach the invented 2.85mmol/L level because parathyroid disease, tumour presence, means that calcium levels are out of control, diseased and therefore unpredictable.

These patients all still require access to surgery without having to do months of research, write letter after letter of complaint or continually fight for their right to life. It can be argued that failure to ensure that all patients with consistently abnormal serum calcium levels are considered for surgery (without any monitoring or weighing up of calcium levels), particularly in light of the above, would be a breach of the Human Rights of patients, in terms of their right to life and protection from neglect. No mythical, and wholly unreasonable, "cut-off" should be included in the guidelines. In fact, in order to ensure that practitioners do not continue to consider the figure of >2.85mmol/L in any of their musings over best practice (which inclusion of this figure is likely to maintain), the guidelines must explicitly explain that the height of abnormal serum calcium has no bearing on whether a patient should be referred for surgery nor is it an indication of number or size of adenomas or severity of symptoms.

It has been noted that Committee Membership at the time the guidelines were introduced consisted of 9 out of 14 people for whom there was a direct potential for financial benefit for ensuring patients remained sick with parathyroid disease. Out of these 9, only 1 committee member who benefits financially (has a private practice) was not allowed to declare or participate in meetings but could answer questions. (EG Q: Shall we include the made-up figure of 2.85? A: Yeah, why not hey?) This must therefore affect the information in the guidance document. There are a number of Hyperparathyroid UK group members who have had no alternative but to seek costly, private consultations and treatment for parathyroid disease, predominantly due to the current vast gaps in knowledge of GPs, endocrinologists and surgeons and the severity of their symptoms, which were not necessarily the prerequisite osteoporosis/kidney disease requirements. It is clearly important that any future guidance and NHS training centres solely on patient/clinical evidence. Patients are not motivated by financial gain, but are the actual people this disease has affected.

In sum, my whole experience with this disease, the absence of any accurate knowledge or awareness of this disease within the medical profession in the UK, the lack of any knowledge of the actual symptoms and the detrimental impact these have on the lives of patients, the lack of compassion and understanding exhibited by many medical professions towards patients suffering (I was told to compare myself to cancer patients on the waiting list for surgery, which I found inappropriate and unfair since these are two wholly different diseases – does a stage 2 cancer patient get asked to compare themselves to someone with stage 4 cancer?) and the prolonged delays in getting treatment/surgery was horrendous. I then predictably didn't receive the 12 month follow up/monitoring appointment, which is necessary post-op and due to my terrible experiences I was reluctant to pursue and battle any more. I waited for 2 years without any contact and once again had to instigate a request for a follow-up. More of the same endless chasing and asking and emailing has therefore resumed. The aftermath in the last 2 years post-surgery has been difficult and particularly affected my mental health and well-being. My experience has left me with anxiety akin to that associated with Post Traumatic Stress Disorder (PTSD). No one should have to have experienced this disease along with the battle against the medical professionals, who are there supposedly to assist. There has been no comeback on the medical professionals who got my diagnosis wrong, who made inaccurate assessments of my symptoms, who treated me with total disregard and neglect and who delayed my treatment due to their lack of knowledge and due to the excrement within the NICE guidelines. There is no accountability for prolonging my suffering, for disregarding my symptoms or for putting my health at greater risk and nothing has changed for the thousands of other patients who will likely suffer the same experiences. I am unable to trust the NHS or medical professionals, and most definitely not NICE and their wholly inaccurate guidelines that risk the health and lives of countless people.

It speaks volumes that I am again fighting against the NHS and NICE and having to write yet another letter. But I feel that anyone else who is left a sick, suicidal wreck as I was, should have someone fighting their corner. Any other course of action would be inhumane.

I trust you will look into this matter as a matter of urgency and I look forward to your response.

Yours sincerely

Mrs Susan Williams

Suzy Langdon

With ref to SJP/SS-CEONHS/15.03.21

Re action needed by NHS England for recognition and treatment of Hyperparathyroidism

Dear Sir Simon Stevens

I am writing with reference to the above to explain my story of hyperparathyroidism.

In 2004 it was discovered that I had raised calcium. I was under the care of an endocrinologist due to a pituitary tumour from 1989. My calcium was monitored for the next fifteen years but no further tests or treatment offered. In 2013 it was discovered that I had Osteopenia. I asked for confirmation of hyperparathyroidism via a scan, only to be told nothing would be done until I had osteoporosis, which I now have.

I cannot understand why investigations and treatment would be withheld until my bones are brittle and likely to cause fractures, hospital stays, and money spent on recuperation. High calcium causes lots of other damage to my body that will diminish my quality of life as well as cost the NHS money that could be saved if treatment was forthcoming a lot earlier. The NICE guidelines do not say wait and see until the patient has a diminished quality of life and it is very unnecessary for this to happen. Many endocrinologist still need educating as to this fact and this is what this letter is all about.

Thanks to the Hyperparathyroid UK Action4Change website and Facebook site I have now recently had surgery from Mr Shad khan in Oxford. He said that I should also have been offered genetic testing due to my age when I was diagnosed with the pituitary tumour in 1989 and Hyperparathyroidism in 2013. My own local endocrinologist told me years ago he was reluctant to send me for this as it was expensive!

I hope that you will be willing to take my point seriously because I am not the only person by a long way. There are hundreds if not thousands of other people who are suffering unnecessarily and unfairly.

Yours sincerely

Mrs Suzy Langdon

Tara Sullivan

Our Ref: SJP/SS-CEO NHS/15-03-21

Dear Sir Simon Stevens

Re: Letter from Sallie Powell, here is my NHS PHPT story.

I am writing to you as a member of Hyperparathyroid UK
Action4Change; I first went to my GP in the summer of 2018 because
I had a slight swelling to the front right side of my neck that hadn't
changed for some months. I had actually felt unwell for years but
dismissed it until the neck swelling appeared. The GP referred me
for a neck ultrasound and to an endocrinologist. Unfortunately the
wait through the NHS was at least twenty eight weeks, but there
were no appointments available so I was unable to book an
Endocrine appointment online. I am a civil servant for the
Metropolitan Police Service and I pay into Benenden Health, so I
asked to be referred to an endocrinologist at Benenden to speed up
the process. A neck ultrasound identified the following;

- Possible parathyroid adenoma
- Developing Thyroiditis (auto antibody results recommended
- Thyroid nodules 5mm-2.4cm in size causing goitre (neck swelling)

A blood Test revealed PTH high at 14 (1.6-7.2), and calcium
low/normal at 2.3 (2.2-2.6)

Benenden endocrinologist requested a myeloma blood test, I was
told results would be available from my GP within 3-4 days. I rang
the results line at my GP surgery every afternoon for over 3 weeks, I
was on the phone for between thirty minutes to over an hour each
day and each day I was told no myeloma results had been received
and to call back the next day. As you can only imagine the anxiety
caused by calling for blood cancer results for 3 weeks. It was only
when I asked to speak to the practice manager that it was discovered
the GP surgery had my result the entire time but the lab called it
Electrophoresis instead of Myeloma. I knew it had been sent

because I called the blood testing clinic, the lab at the hospital myself, and they informed me that the results had been sent to my GP surgery more than once but they could not tell me the result. Thankfully this was a normal result.

In February 2019, a kidney ultrasound reported the following;

- Right 93mm / Left 99mm
- Bilaterally moderate cortical thickness
- Negligible post micturition residual is imaged

A sestamibi scan reported no evidence of an adenoma, but to consider parathyroid hyperplasia. A DEXA bone density scan was normal. In March, my vitamin D was found to be very low at 12 (30-200), and a 24hr urine calcium test revealed 2.1 low output (2.50-7.50mmol/24hrs). The endocrinologist diagnosed secondary hyperparathyroidism.

Unfortunately, the Benenden time-frame is 6-months, so all of my tests were done between December 2018-March 2019 after that you cannot be referred for the same ailment within two years, so I had lots of results but no treatment and I was referred back to my GP just as my vitamin D deficiency was discovered.

My GP called me at work immediately prescribing a high dose of D for 3-months 20,000 IU, daily for 14 days, then 1 tablet each fortnight for further 10-wks. Then I was given another blood test form to have done once course of tablets was finished.

June 19 Blood Test; PTH normal at 3.8 (1.60-6.90 pmol/L), Calcium 2.4 (2.2-2.6). *Vitamin D was not retested as it was within 6 months of previous test.*

I have an identical twin sister who has similar blood results to me; she suffers from dilated cardiomyopathy which was the result of a virus in 2001. More recently, she has suffered from a heart attack and a stroke from the damage the virus caused and had an ICD implanted in September 2019. It was suggested that I should have my heart screened.

11/07/19 ECG: Abnormality consider anteroseptal myocardial symptoms.

Note: Secondary Hyperparathyroidism causes cardiovascular complications & abnormal fat and sugar metabolism

I felt another lump on my neck so visited the GP who sent me for another ultrasound in summer 2019 which located two possible adenomas. The GP recommended an urgent ENT referral was needed. At the ENT appointment I was told the nodules were benign, throat unobstructed, however the possible adenomas were not mentioned at all, even though they were the reason for my referral. ENT ordered another blood test & MRI. I gave them copies of all my previous test results and scans from Benenden, which were not in my NHS file.

In November ENT said the MRI confirmed the nodules were benign. As my thyroid was ok; despite having numerous thyroid nodules and thyroiditis, I was told I was being transferred to another doctor who had reviewed my notes and wanted to do a biopsy, and that I would receive an appointment letter in post. In my hospital notes it shows that ENT referred me in October 2019 by but a biopsy was not written in my hospital notes.

I was very ill with Covid symptoms for over 7 weeks during March 2020 and April 2020 so I isolated as per government guidelines at the time. Covid tests were not available at this time as it was early in the Pandemic. An appointment with an endocrinologist was changed to a telephone appointment due to Covid. After a five month wait for this appointment, the doctor was very rude and dismissive when I described my symptoms he said that they could not be related and only became interested when I said I was due to see a surgeon on 02/04/20. I received another appt to see him on October 2020. The appointment with the surgeon was cancelled.

In August 2020 I received letters discharging me from both doctors without seeing either of them. Two years on, no treatment, none of my results have ever been discussed with me, I have not had a biopsy of the suspicious growths that were seen in every ultrasound from December 2018, which causes me great concern.

I posted my journey on "Hyperparathyroid UK's medical group HPT UK Medical and spoke to Mr Shad Khan, Endocrine Surgeon at Oxford University Hospitals; Shahab.khan@ouh.nhs.uk . He said he would like to help if my GP would refer me to him. I have spoken to him a couple of times in the last few months, he has restored my faith in the NHS, he listens and I felt validated for the first time since this all started. Most of my tests were over a year old so he wrote to my GP requesting more tests.

10/02/21 PET Choline scan at Churchill Hospital in Oxford; Mr Khan called me afterwards to tell me that there is definitely something lighting up in my scan that needs further investigation and that once my other tests were done he would book me in for surgery. A blood Test and neck ultrasound were requested. My calcium has never been high, so my concern is the growths/tumours that have been seen in every ultrasound scan. I have had many different diagnoses over the past 2 & ½ years; secondary hyperparathyroid, thyroid nodules, thyroiditis, parathyroid adenomas (although I have been told I do not have primary PHPT), vitamin D deficiency and more recently my kidneys do not appear to be functioning well.

I have many symptoms; massive weight gain, despite suffering from loose stools for approx. 6yrs, Insomnia, fatigue, muscle and bone pain, blurred vision, dizziness, restless legs, tingling hands and numbness, anxiety, depression, goitre, neck pain, kidney pain, heart palpitations, heartburn, tinnitus. I am unable to kneel, as it is too painful.

It seems that information relating to secondary hyperparathyroidism, normocalcemic PHPT and normohormonal PHPT require further study and recognition within the NHS, there are studies in America that were published over twenty years ago. Unfortunately the reality is that NHS patients have no entitlement to a parathyroidectomy unless they have high calcium levels, kidney stones or osteoporosis, so like myself are being discharged when they are still suffering.

My life has changed greatly as a result of this illness, as mentioned I work for the Police Service but I have felt unable to increase to full-time hours as my children have grown older for health reasons. I previously volunteered as a Cub Scout Leader, responsible for looking after twenty six x 8-10yr olds, which I had to give up due to my poor health. I am currently waiting for a surgery date with Mr Khan.

Please look at the following website: Hyperparathyroiduk.com

NICE guideline; https://www.nice.org.uk/guidance/NG132

Regards

Mrs Tara Sullivan

Vicky Haynes

Professor Amanda Howe RCGP President

Dear Professor Howe,

ONE PATIENT'S JOURNEY

Re: Campaign for radical improvement in GP's understanding, recognition and treatment of Primary Hyperparathyroidism

Reference: Hyperparathyroid UK letter ref SJP/AH-RCGP/15-03-21

I am writing to you in support for Hyperparathyroid UK's campaign for the better recognition and treatment of Primary Hyperparathyroidism (PHPT).

Hyperparathyroidism is a disease few doctors appear to really understand. It is not surprising therefore that it is one of the most commonly undiagnosed illnesses in the UK. Even when it is diagnosed, doctors often recommend a watch and wait approach when it is known that this is a degenerative disease for which the only known cure is minor surgery. The NHS could save millions by prompt surgical removal of a rogue gland that has developed into a benign adenoma. Occasionally more than one gland is affected. The patient's journey starts with their GP.

Patients often present with varying symptoms from aching bones to unimaginable tiredness and so many more symptoms. The disease is often misdiagnosed as fibromyalgia or poly myalgia, depression, menopause or even hypochondria! It affects every cell in your body and is totally destructive. Calcium at elevated levels is a poison and eventually, if the disease is not addressed, can kill you. The NHS spends a fortune treating the consequences of hyperparathyroidism and not the cause.

In May 2019, after considerable encouragement from Hyperparathyroid UK and others, NICE issued guidelines for the diagnosis, assessment and initial management of PHPT. Hyperparathyroid UK believes there are serious shortcomings in these NICE guidelines as currently written, principally that they do not adequately address normocalcemic HPT or normohormonal HPT. However, in my personal experience GP's are generally ignorant of the current guidelines.

My personal journey was tough and at times frightening. For years my bloods showed elevated blood calcium levels. I also had symptoms of kidney disease and heart arrhythmia. I saw both renal and cardiology consultants but none pursued high calcium despite kidney damage and flecks of calcium being seen in my aorta. More recently my bloods started to show elevated ALP indicating high bone turnover. My GP was concerned that the ALP might point towards bone cancer. She instigated a deeper investigation which fortunately included a blood test for vitamin D level.

My husband, who is an Engineer, put the concurrent symptoms of raised calcium and low vitamin D into an internet search. The search indicated a high probability of PHPT. Further internet searching confirmed that PHPT often causes elevated ALP. It also led to Hyperparathyroid UK's website that stressed the importance of testing for parathyroid hormone (PTH) in accordance with the NICE guidelines. I then had a bit of battle with my GP to get my PTH tested correctly. I had to quote the NICE guidelines and insist that they were followed. This confirmed elevated calcium and PTH. I was referred to an endocrinologist who was not convinced and voiced the opinion that I didn't have PHPT. He said he would test for ionised calcium to confirm his opinion. The result confounded his opinion and confirmed I had PHPT. However, he thought it was "mild" and said I could watch and wait.
I insisted on being referred to a surgeon (see NICE Guidelines para 1.3.2).

In the surgeon, I finally met the first medical practitioner who appeared to understand the disease. She said I had elevated calcium, elevated parathyroid hormone and was symptomatic. In September 2020, she performed a parathyroidectomy on me, removing one enlarged gland. Histology confirmed it was an adenoma. All my blood levels, calcium, PTH and ALP immediately returned to within normal range. I am cured of hyperparathyroidism, all my related symptoms have dissipated and I have felt so much better ever since.

I urge you as President of the Royal Society of General Practitioners to address the general lack of understanding of hyperparathyroidism and champion an update to the NICE Guidelines in the interest of patients and of the NHS.

Thank you for taking the time to read all our letters and hopefully we can have a resolution and move forward with diagnosis and treatments.

Yours sincerely,

Vicky Haynes

Courtesy copy sent to my GP Practice

W T

Our Ref: SJP/AH-RCGP/15-03-21

Dear Amanda

I am writing in support of the campaign organised by the Founder/CEO of Hyperparathyroid UK Action4Change, relating to the misdiagnosis and mistreatment of Primary Hyperparathyroidism in the UK. My story is mainly related to the lack of appropriate treatment from the consultants at my NHS Trust, but I do have to question why it took seven years for my GP surgery to request the appropriate tests that would have confirmed my diagnosis earlier.

I have felt unwell for a long time, with joint and bone pain, and other symptoms that I can now relate to my diagnosis of Primary Hyperparathyroidism. In fact, I can see from my GP notes that my blood calcium level has been raised, and my kidney function mildly impaired since at least 2013 but despite more visits to the GP nobody noticed or investigated further. In 2019 I sought the advice of a different GP and this time she spotted the signs of hyperparathyroidism. I was referred to an endocrinologist and was given a diagnosis of possible PHPT. However, my symptoms and blood results were dismissed as mild, and as I don't appear to have osteoporosis or serious kidney disease, I was told that surgery would be a drastic solution seeing as I didn't seem that ill. In later appointments, I was told surgery might be required but it might not cure my symptoms. Scans eventually showed I do have parathyroid adenomas and so the only resolution is surgery but now the surgeon is not following the NICE guidelines. The proposal is for an operation on one side instead of the recommended four gland exploration indicated by the scan results and a further surgery if it does not cure me, which is contrary to the NICE guidelines.

The only cure for hyperparathyroidism is surgery but too many endocrinologists adopt a 'watch and wait' practice that only results in damage to bones and kidneys and prolonged suffering for patients. In my own case, I feel compelled to seek a second opinion to obtain the correct treatment and even to consider proceeding with my treatment privately as the NHS seems unable or unwilling to provide the appropriate treatment I require.

In the meantime, I continue to suffer the impact of my illness to my life. Owing to fatigue and pain, I can no longer enjoy the exercise and dance classes that I used to. I am unable to walk for any length of time, climbing the stairs is a challenge and I am in pain and discomfort all the time, all of which can only have a detrimental effect on my wellbeing.

Please give your urgent consideration to the issues raised by Sallie and the members of the group particularly in respect of more training for GPs in respect of Primary Hyperparathyroidism.

Yours sincerely,

WT

Responses to our letters

Responses to our letters so far, have been few and far between. Of course, we understand the effect of Covid-19 on the NHS. The majority of operations in our group were cancelled for thirteen months. As we are lead to believe, Covid will be staying with us for the foreseeable future, so as we already postponed this event by two months, we decided to go ahead in March. As you will have seen, most of our members have not only been affected in the last thirteen months, but for decades.

Andrew Goodall CEO of NHS Wales was very quick to respond. He wrote a very courteous letter forwarded to me within a few days. Sadly, though, he concluded with;

'Hyperparathyroidism is a common condition and I am advised that diagnosis is not a complicated clinical process. I do not believe there is currently a robust enough case for nationally-led healthcare professional education on the diagnosis and management of hyperparathyroidism or for greater specialisation among the endocrinologist community'

I replied;

'Dear Sarah,

Would you please thank Andrew Goodall on my behalf for responding so promptly to my letter of 15th March 2021, and please pass my response to him? He suggested that we contact NICE directly regarding an update to the guidelines for primary hyperparathyroidism. As we know from previous experience, guideline updates have to be commissioned by NHS England, or RCGP. It was our efforts as a group that succeeded in getting the guidelines commissioned originally by RCGP.

I wrote to Professor Amanda Howe, and the CEOs in England,

Scotland, Ireland, and Northern Ireland also on 15th March as we have members in all these areas who have been fighting for a diagnosis for several years. We certainly have a good number of those members in Wales, with a number who have had to pay privately to get surgery in England after struggling to get surgery or even a diagnosis, in Wales. This obviously should not be the case.

As Mr. Goodall wrote in his letter, 'Hyperparathyroidism is a common condition and I am advised that diagnosis is not a complicated clinical process', a problem in Wales appears to be the denial of hyperparathyroidism in any classification other than hypercalcemic primary hyperparathyroidism. Patients with normocalcemic primary hyperparathyroidism are denied surgery in Wales, despite much evidence indicating osteoporosis, kidney stones, and cardiac disease is often presented in normocalcemic patients. Consequently, patients with normocalcemic primary hyperparathyroidism, including those with hyperplasia, MEN1, and also quite a number whose calcium has previously been considerably high, but fallen back into the normal range (which can happen as levels fluctuate with PHPT), are being refused the cure they are entitled to.

The reason we wrote to NHS CEOs, is because we believe they remain unaware of the reality below them in clinical practice. We currently have 2,100 members in our main support group, and over 500 in our medical group HPT UK Medical, The medical group is for medical people who wish to see for themselves the extent of people suffering prolonged mismanagement of this disease. Andrew Goodall would be very welcome to join us to see for himself the reality, as well as see surgical evidence of large adenomas removed from normocalcemic patients.

I will be publishing a book this weekend called One Hundred Letters, which is a collection of heartfelt letters written on 15th March detailing why we have decided to ask for help to stop the unnecessary suffering of mismanaged primary hyperparathyroidism. I am also working on a book about normocalcemic primary hyperparathyroidism in the UK. I hope Andrew Goodall might be interested to read both of them'

Kind regards

Sallie Powell
hyperparathyroiduk.com

A handful of us received a brief acknowledgement for our letters from both RCGP and NHS England. I received this response from NHS England on 22nd March:

'Dear Customer,

Thank you for your email. We are currently receiving a higher than usual volume of emails so it may take us a little longer to respond directly to your email. In the meantime, you may find the following information helpful.

Please note: our normal working hours are 08:00 to 18:00 from Monday to Friday (excluding Bank Holidays). Emails received at the weekend will not be reviewed until the next working day.'

I sent a typed letter to Professor Amanda Howe and a copy by email to Professor Amanda Howe. I received the following response by email on the 17th March;

'Dear Miss Powell
Thank you for your email.
It is receiving our attention.
Kind regards'

There was a slightly more comprehensive response to one member

Thank you for your email to Simon. We have received this and I will pass it on to the team that are developing a response.

We aim to respond to yourself and fellow members very soon.

Best wishes

Another member received this further reply;

'My sincere apologies. I can confirm receipt of a number of emails and letters on this subject. We have commissioned the appropriate team to look into this and provide a response, which I expect in due course. I'm afraid that we were receiving a far higher volume of correspondence addressed to Simon than usual, with many of our team still deployed on Covid work. As such, I'm unable to confirm receipt to everyone but please do share with your network that we are aware and speaking to colleagues about this.

We will endeavour to respond to everyone very soon. Thank you for your patience in the meantime.

Best wishes'

We remain hopeful that NHS England will give serious consideration to our letters and take necessary and long overdue action to help patients with all **four** biochemical classifications of primary hyperparathyroidism. But as of this second edition on 10 may 2021, we have yet to receive any responses from NHS England, Scotland, Ireland, or Northern Ireland.

I received a very courteous response from Dr Jonathan Leach OBE on Friday 24 April, on behalf of Professor Amanda Howe, saying he will ensure my concerns and those of others, are forwarded to the NICE team at their next quarterly meeting with RCGP. He also wrote that Dr Jawaid's (a member of the Expert Committee which developed the NICE guideline along with other stakeholders invited by NICE) article 'Hyperparathyroidism (Primary) NICE guideline; diagnosis, assessment and initial management' was published in the British Journal of General practitioners on 25 January 2020 and that the BJGP is circulated to all 54,000 members of RCGP. I haven't seen the article, but I can only assume either a vast number of those members missed or failed to understand the article.

Whether they missed it or failed to understand it, they have a duty of care to their patients, which many of them are failing to uphold.

Dr Jonathan Leach OBE has informed me twice now about this article, implying that it should have been enough to educate 54000 GPs on current practice for the recognition, and appropriate treatment and referral processes for primary hyperparathyroidism.

Quite obviously, the seventy eight letters in this book, show more action is required, with some urgency. That was after all, the purpose of writing the letters. They are a small fraction of the amount of similar cases. We have over 2200 current members with very similar stories.

One of our members Sue Mckinny, contacted The UK Society of Endocrinology on 11 April 2021 about misinformation on their site, as mentioned in our introduction. We were most impressed to hear she had the following response on the 7 May.

Dear Sue,

Many thanks for contacting 'You and Your Hormones.'

We passed your query to the Editorial Board, who have reviewed this section and altered the wording to be clearer and more accurate. It is very useful to have patient input for continual improvement of the website content that better informs people on hormones and health.

Here is their amended and more accurate entry;

If hypercalcaemia is caused by primary hyperparathyroidism, it is important to treat this condition in order to improve symptoms and prevent long-term problems such as osteoporosis or kidney stones. Primary hyperparathyroidism requires an early specialist opinion to determine if symptoms are related to the hyperparathyroidism. Expertise is required to identify whether a parathyroid swelling (adenoma) is present before surgical removal. If an adenoma is identified, the aims of surgical removal are reversal of symptoms, prevention of long-term complications and normalisation of calcium levels. In patients where an operation is not possible, specialist medication may be needed to lower parathyroid hormone levels.

Coming soon from Sallie Powell...

A modern day medical mystery; The medical denial of normocalcemic primary hyperparathyroidism (NCPHPT) in the UK;

Normocalcemic PHPT has been recognised and talked about in America for twenty five years. It has been talked about in medical studies in the UK since 1948! Yet there are surgeons in the UK who claim 'Normocalcemic is not even a thing'. There are surgeons who refuse to recognise it, and who refuse to operate, even with a positive localisation scan.

There are many conflicting medical articles/studies describing Normocalcemic Primary Hyperparathyroidism as; a 'new phase', a 'mild phase of PHPT, a 'newly recognised phase', a 'precursor to hypercalcemic primary hyperparathyroidism'. We believe it has always been there.

There are also many medical studies describing NCPHPT patients as being more likely to suffer with osteoporosis, kidney stones, and heart disease. It makes perfect sense to members of Hyperparathyroid UK Action4Change that these patients have been left undiagnosed for years to be affected so severely. Yet, still they are denied a diagnosis or the same cure as hypercalcemic patients, a parathyroidectomy.

A Modern Day Medical Mystery will set the record straight about Normocalcemic Primary Hyperparathyroidism, providing decades of evidence alongside modern day case stories of people who have had surgery performed by the few surgeons in the UK who don't dismiss the need for surgery. We have pictures of large adenomas removed from normocalcemic patients by respected surgeons, and wonderful stories of a return to great health after surgery.

For more information about Hyperparathyroid UK Action4Change, please visit our website which is a valuable tool for people who suspect PHPT, or want to know more about it; hyperparathyroiduk.com or follow Sallie Powell on Twitter; @SpSallie

About HPT UK

Hyperparathyroid UK Action4Change is a Patient to Patient support group on Facebook. We all have the same goal. We all want to have the parathyroid disease removed that is holding our body and mind to ransom.

We don't deserve to lose our family and friends, who tire of us fighting for a diagnosis that our doctors don't understand, to be known unfairly as hypochondriacs, or to have our physical symptoms wrongly blamed on depression, lifestyle, or age.

We don't want to be forced year upon year to keep going back to poorly educated doctors pleading for referrals or scans when our biological results clearly show we have PHPT.

We don't want to 'watch and wait' while PHPT takes a hold of our body and mind. We don't want to wake up in pain and go to bed in pain knowing from the experience of hundreds of others, that some, if not all of our symptoms can be alleviated by surgery. We don't want to be forced to lose our jobs whilst our doctors dither over whether or not to refer us or to review us in 12 months. We don't want to endure the humiliation forced on us by those same doctors.

If you are reading this book and think you know somebody who may have undiagnosed primary hyperparathyroidism, please refer them to our website.

If you are an endocrinologist, GP, surgeon or medical student, with an interest in primary hyperparathyroidism, and would like to join our medical group, in a private setting on Facebook, please send us a request to join HPT UK Medical

Printed in Great Britain
by Amazon

22898345R00149